Forging Links
for Health Research

Forging Links *for* Health Research

Perspectives from the Council on Health Research for Development

EDITED BY VICTOR NEUFELD AND NANCY JOHNSON

INTERNATIONAL DEVELOPMENT RESEARCH CENTRE
Ottawa • Cairo • Dakar • Johannesburg • Montevideo • Nairobi • New Delhi • Singapore

© International Development Research Centre 2001

Published by the International Development Research Centre
PO Box 8500, Ottawa, ON, Canada K1G 3H9
http://www.idrc.ca

Canadian Cataloging in Publication Data

Main entry under title :

Forging links for health research : perspectives from the Council on Health Research for Development

Includes bibliographical references.
ISBN 0-88936-935-6

1. Public health — Research — Developing countries.
2. Medical care — Research — Developing countries.
3. Public health — Developing countries.
4. Medical care — Developing countries.
I. Neufeld, Victor.
II. Johnson, Nancy.
III. Council on Health Research for Development.
IV. International Development Research Centre (Canada)

RA441.5F67 2000   362.1'07'21724   C00-980454-4

All rights reserved. No part of this publication may be reproduced, stored in a retrieval system, or transmitted, in any form or by any means, electronic, mechanical, photocopying, or otherwise, without the prior permission of the International Development Research Centre. Mention of a proprietary name does not constitute endorsement of the product and is given only for information. A microfiche edition is available.

IDRC Books endeavours to produce environmentally friendly publications. All paper used is recycled as well as recyclable. All inks and coatings are vegetable-based products.

CONTENTS

Preface — *Charas Suwanwela and Yvo Nuyens* vii

Acknowledgments — *Victor Neufeld and Nancy Johnson* ix

PART I: HEALTH, EQUITY, AND RESEARCH

Chapter 1.   Meeting the Challenge: A Decade of Activity 3
— *Victor Neufeld and Nancy Johnson*

Chapter 2.   Health for Some: Health, Poverty, and Equity
at the Beginning of the 21st Century 29
— *Tessa Tan-Torres Edejer*

Chapter 3.   Health Research: An Essential Tool for
Achieving Development Through Equity 47
— *David Harrison*

PART II: PUTTING COUNTRIES FIRST

Chapter 4.   Community Participation in Essential
National Health Research 81
— *Susan Reynolds Whyte*

Chapter 5.   Linking Research to Policy and Action 109
— *Somsak Chunharas*

Chapter 6.   Fostering a National Capacity for
Equity-oriented Health Research 141
— *Victor Neufeld*

Chapter 7. Regional Perspectives 179
— *Javid Hashmi, Tamas Koos, Peter Makara,
Abdelhay Mechbal, Mutuma Mugambi,
Victor Neufeld, Alberto Pellegrini Filho,
David Picou, and Chitr Sitthi-amorn*

PART III: THE WAY AHEAD

Chapter 8. COHRED and ENHR: An Update
and Look Ahead 213
— *Yvo Nuyens, Charas Suwanwela,
and Nancy Johnson*

Chapter 9. Health Research for Development:
Realities and Challenges 241
— *Charas Suwanwela and Victor Neufeld*

Appendix 1. Contributing Authors 267

Appendix 2. Abbreviations and Acronyms 273

Appendix 3. Bibliography 277

PREFACE

This book looks at the contribution of health research to development and, in particular, the equity dimension of development. Its title, *Forging Links for Health Research*, is a reference to the 1990 report of the Commission on Health Research for Development, *Health Research: Essential Link to Equity in Development*. In this report, the Commission asserted that research has the power to "enable developing countries to strengthen health action and to discover new and more effective means to deal with unsolved health problems" (CHRD 1990, p. xix). It also reflected on the need for stronger links between all stakeholders in the health-research process, if it is to be truly an integral part of development.

The Commission established the Council on Health Research for Development (COHRED) to work with developing countries in implementing the Essential National Health Research (ENHR) strategy, which aims at furthering equity in health development. COHRED offers technical support to enable countries to implement ENHR and works with national research leaders to promote health research as a tool for development, establish research priorities, strengthen mechanisms to support research, and build research and user capacities. COHRED also works to bring about interaction between leaders in health research, within and between countries, so that these countries can share experiences and insights on the implementation of the ENHR strategy.

This volume presents the views and experiences of a number of individuals, groups, and institutions involved in ENHR over the past decade. It highlights the key achievements, as well as the setbacks, since the 1990s and the prospects for health research in the coming decades. The book has three parts. The first of these has three chapters. Chapter 1 gives an account of the main events of the past decade in health research for development. Chapter 2 is an essay on the evolving understanding of inequities in health. Chapter 3 offers an analysis of the contribution of health research to human development.

Part II focuses mainly on the country experience of three aspects of the health-research process: promoting community participation (Chapter 4), translating research into action and policy (Chapter 5), and strengthening the capacities of national health-research systems (Chapter 6). Chapter 7 then gives "snapshots" of the health-research situation in several regions and provides an analysis of the contribution of regional arrangements to national health-research efforts. The final part looks to the future. It has two chapters. Chapter 8 tells the COHRED story, including its efforts to assess its own contributions and find ways to meet future challenges. This chapter also presents the views of national health-research leaders from developing countries. The final chapter summarizes important realities confronting the global health-research community at the beginning of the new century and presents key challenges for those responsible for national health-research systems, especially those committed to making health research a stronger tool for equitable health development.

As indicated in the list of authors in Appendix 1 and in the acknowledgments below, this book was a collaborative effort of many individuals, particularly those from low- to middle-income countries. Most chapters are the result of a participatory writing process, in which a group of colleagues provided feedback to one or more lead writers. As well, health-research leaders in a number of developing countries contributed their views on the way ahead, through a series of in-depth interviews.

The book thus combines a look into the mirror of the past with an attempt to gaze into the crystal ball of what lies ahead. In other words, it uses reflections from the past to take us forward into the uncharted territory of the future. We hope that it will contribute to the continuing dialogue between all involved travelers and help steer the journey toward more equitable health development.

Charas Suwanwela
Chair, COHRED Board

Yvo Nuyens
COHRED Coordinator

ACKNOWLEDGMENTS

This book was a collaborative project involving many persons in addition to the authors. We gratefully acknowledge the wisdom and assistance of the following individuals. For any omissions or errors in this list, we apologize.

Mohamed Said Abdullah
National Health Research and
 Development Centre, Kenya

Gopal Prasad Acharya
Nepal Health Research Council,
 Nepal

Joselito Acuin
De La Salle University, Philippines

Sam Adjei
Health Research Unit
Ministry of Health, Ghana

Aikan Akanov
National Health Lifestyle Centre,
 Kazakhstan

Tasleem Akhtar
Provincial Health Services Academy
Northwest Frontier Province,
 Pakistan

Bienvenido Alana
Centre for Economic Policy
 Research, Philippines

Eusebbe Alihonou
Regional Centre for Health and
 Development, Benin

Celia Almeida
Network for Health Systems and
 Services Research
Oswaldo Cruz Foundation, Brazil

Said Ameerberg
Mauritius Institute of Health,
 Mauritius

Asuncion Anden
Tuklas Pangkalusugan Foundation
Essential National Health Research
 Program
Department of Health, Philippines

Isao Arita
Agency for Cooperation in
 International Health, Japan

Hilda Bastian
Cochrane Collaboration Consumer
 Network, Australia

Dennis Batangan
Tuklas Pangkalusugan Foundation
Essential National Health Research
 Program
Department of Health, Philippines

Boungnong Bhoupa
Council of Medical Sciences
Ministry of Health, Lao PDR

Abbas Bhuiya
International Centre for Diarrheal
  Disease Research, Bangladesh

Robert Chambers
Institute of Development Studies,
  United Kingdom

Steve Chandiwana
Ministry of Health and Child
  Welfare
Blair Research Institute, Zimbabwe

Abu Yusuf Choudhury
Program for the Introduction and
  Adaptation of Contraceptive
  Technology, Bangladesh

Peter Czerny
Canadian Society for International
  Health, Canada

Sylvia Dehaan
Council on Health Research
  for Development, Geneva,
  Switzerland

Don de Savigny
International Development
  Research Centre, Tanzania

Alpha Amadou Diallo
Ministry of Public Health, Guinea

F. Binta Diallo
Consultant, Guinea

Pham Huy Dung
Centre for Social Science Research
  for Health
Ministry of Health, Viet Nam

Patrick Okello Emegu
Makerere Medical School, Uganda

E.M. Essien
Haematology Department
University of Ibadan, Nigeria

John Evans
Torstar Corporation, Canada

Mario Festin
University of the Philippines
  (Manila), Philippines

Norbert Forster
Ministry of Health and Child
  Welfare, Namibia

Claudette Francis
Clinical Psychologist, Consultant,
  Trinidad

Lucinda Franklin
Council on Health Research for
  Development, South Africa

Lennart Friej
Council on Health Research for
  Development, Geneva,
  Switzerland

Ansgar Gerhardus
Department of Tropical Hygiene
  and Public Health
University of Heidelberg, Germany

Izzy Gerstenbluth
Department of Epidemiology and
  Research
Medical and Public Health Service
  of Curaçau, Curaçao

Vilius Grabauskas
Kaunas Medical University,
  Lithuania

Samia Yousif Idris Habbani
Research Directorate
Federal Ministry of Health, Sudan

Jan Hatcher-Roberts
Canadian Society for International
  Health, Canada

Manikavasagam Jegathesan
Malaysia

Matthias Kerker
Council on Health Research for
  Development, Geneva,
  Switzerland

Andrew Kitua
National Institute for Medical
  Research, Tanzania

Mary Ann Lansang
University of the Philippines
  (Manila), Philippines

Adetokunbo Lucas
Independent Consultant, London,
  United Kingdom

Peter Makara
World Health Organization
Regional Office for Europe,
  Copenhagen, Denmark

Angelito Manalili
College of Social Work and
  Community Development
University of the Philippines
  (Manila), Philippines

Adolfo Martínez-Palomo
Centro de Investigación y de
  Estudios Avanzados Del Instituto
  Politécnio Nacional, Mexico

Laura McDougall
Public Health and Primary Care
  Unit
University of the West Indies,
  St Augustine, Trinidad

Cary Miller
United States Agency for International Development, United States

Hanne Mogensen
Institute of Anthropology
University of Copenhagen,
  Denmark

Rajanenath Mohabeer
Ministry of Health, Mauritius

Fernando Munoz
Latin America Centre for the Study
  of Health Systems, Chile

Francisco Muzio
Project for Foot and Mouth Disease
  Control and Eradication in the
  River Plate Basin
Pan American Foot-and-Mouth
  Disease Center
Pan American Health Organization,
  Washington, DC, United States

Stella Neema
Makerere Institute of Social
  Research, Makerere University,
  Uganda

Soumare Absatou N'iaye
Community Health Department,
  Mali

David Okello
World Health Organization
Regional Office for Africa
Harare, Zimbabwe

Greit Onsea
Council on Health Research for
  Development, Kenya

Raphael Owor
Faculty of Medicine
Makerere University, Uganda

Tikki Pang
World Health Organization
Research Policy and Co-ordination,
  Evidence and Information for
  Policy, Geneva, Switzerland

Michael Phillips
Research Centre of Clinical
  Epidemiology
Beijing Hui Long Guan Hospital,
  China

Kamashwar Prasad
All India Institute of Medical
  Sciences, New Delhi, India

Akhtar Ali Qureshi
Health Services Academy
Ministry of Health, Pakistan

V. Ramalingaswami
All India Institute of Medical Sciences, New Delhi, India

Laurie Ramiro
University of the Philippines (Manila), Philippines

Duangjai Sahassananda
Tropical Medicine and Public Health Center
South East Asian Ministers of Education Organization, Thailand

Bassiouni S. Salem
Upgrading Primary Health Care Services
Ministry of Public Health, Egypt

Roberto Salvatella
Universidad de la República, Montevideo, Uruguay

Delia Sánchez
Grupo de Estudios en Economía Organización y Políticas Sociales, Uruguay

Anita Sandstrom
Swedish International Development Agency, Sweden

Lye Munn Sann
Institute of Medical Research, Malaysia

Eugene Smolensky
University of California at Berkeley, United States

Paing Soe
Ministry of Health, Myanmar

Agus Suwandono
Center for Health Systems Research and Development
Ministry of Health, Indonesia

N'nah Djénab Sylla
Ministry of Public Health, Guinea

Peter Tugwell
University of Ottawa, Canada

Ma. Theresa Ujano-Batangan
Tuklas Pangkalusugan Foundation
Essential National Health Research Program
Department of Health, Philippines

Tissa Vitarana
Ministry of Science Technology and Human Resources Development, Sri Lanka

Steven Wayling
Special Programme for Research and Training in Tropical Diseases
World Health Organization, Geneva, Switzerland

Dennis Willms
McMaster University, Canada

Richard Wilson
France

Victor Neufeld
Nancy Johnson

Part I

Health, Equity, and Research

CHAPTER 1

MEETING THE CHALLENGE: A DECADE OF ACTIVITY

Victor Neufeld and Nancy Johnson

SUMMARY

> *Research uses the scientific method to discover facts and their interrelationships and then to apply this new knowledge in practical settings. This process was the means by which the jet engine was invented, the atom split, and the green revolution of the past 25 years generated. Research holds the same promise for health, a promise that we have seen fulfilled with the development of new tools such as antibiotics for the treatment of disease, vaccines for its prevention, and insecticides for controlling the vectors that transmit it. Yet for the world's most vulnerable people, the benefits of research offer a potential for change that has gone largely untapped.*
> — CHRD (1990, p. vii)

This was the challenge, just more than 12 years ago. It led to a major review by an independent international initiative, the Commission on Health Research for Development, to determine why this was the case and what could be done. After 2 years of intensive consultation and debate, the Commission presented its findings and recommendations to an international conference at the Karolinska Institute in Stockholm, Sweden, in February 1990. Its principal finding was that only 5% of the global health-research investment is directed to conditions accounting for 95% of global disease. It recommended four actions:

— Encourage all countries to undertake Essential National Health Research (ENHR);

— Address common health problems through international partnerships linking the efforts of developing and industrialized countries;

— Mobilize larger and more sustained financial support from international sources to supplement developing-country investments; and

— Establish an international mechanism to monitor progress and promote financial and technical support for research on health problems in developing countries.

A direct follow-up from the Stockholm conference was the interim Task Force on Health Research for Development. It began working with developing countries implementing the ENHR strategy and set the stage for a more permanent mechanism to support their efforts. This was the Council on Health Research for Development (COHRED), a Geneva-based nongovernmental organization (NGO), established in March 1993.

During the 1990s, the World Health Organization (WHO) was also active in strengthening the role of research to address the health problems of the world's needy peoples. An important example was a collaborative analysis of global health-research priorities, resulting in the 1996 report, *Investing in Health Research and Development* (Ad Hoc Committee 1996). In 1993, for the first time, the World Bank's annual world development report focused on health (World Bank 1993). Since then the World Bank has become an increasingly important investor in health development, including health research. Another new institution, the Global Forum for Health Research (GFHR), was created in 1996 to provide a forum for stakeholders to review global health-research priorities, promote ongoing analysis of the international health-research situation, and facilitate coalition-building. The central objective of GFHR is "to help correct the 10/90 gap" (GFHR 1999, p. 8).

This chapter summarizes other examples of efforts to strengthen health research and its application to important national and global health problems, including several international programs: International Clinical Epidemiology Network (INCLEN), International Health Policy Program (IHPP), Applied Research on Child Health (ARCH) project, and the Multilateral Initiative on Malaria (MIM). It also discusses examples of special initiatives in some industrialized countries: the Swedish Agency for Research Cooperation with Developing Countries (SAREC), Canada's International Development Research Centre (IDRC), and the Swiss Commission for Research Partnerships with Developing Countries (SCRPDC).

The chapter concludes with the view that although one finds more awareness of the 10/90 disequilibrium over the past decade and intensified action at national, regional, and global levels, the "system" is still too fragmented and uncoordinated. This raises questions about how effectively global health research has benefited the world's most vulnerable people during this time, which in turn sets the stage for the chapters that follow.

INTRODUCTION

In the last 10–15 years of the 20th century, the international development community made an effort to examine the role of health research as an important contributor to sustainable human development. Leading this endeavour was the work of the independent international Commission on Health Research for Development, which presented its landmark report to the Nobel Conference in Stockholm in February 1990. Several other organizations and agencies have shared its concerns and initiated special programs, including United Nations agencies, principally WHO and the World Bank. These actors have reached considerable agreement about the challenges and possible strategies to address them.

Now, as a new century begins, it is appropriate that the global health research-and-development (R&D) community will be meeting in Bangkok, Thailand, in October 2000. It will review progress on actions recommended a decade ago and renew a vision and an action agenda for the coming years.

Within this context, a group of colleagues concerned about the role of health research as an "essential link" to equity in development produced this document. This book is one among a number of contributions to the global review of health research for development. It attempts primarily to present a national perspective, with a special emphasis on the experiences and views of developing countries. It complements other documents prepared for the international conference, which focus more on global issues, such as the future "architecture" for health-research cooperation or the current status and future prospects for global financial flows.

This background introductory chapter will

— Restate the problems — or challenges — as described 10 years ago;

— Summarize the findings and recommendations of the Commission and trace follow-up actions, with special attention to what has been done to facilitate ENHR in developing countries;

— Highlight the roles and activities of other key players in health R&D over the past decade or so, including WHO, the World Bank, GFHR, some international programs, and some donor countries; and

— Comment on the status of the international health-research system at the beginning of this century, as it addresses the globally dominant health problems of our time.

THE PROBLEM AS SEEN 10 YEARS AGO

Ten years ago, the Commission described the problems and challenges confronting the international health-research community. At the development level, it felt that people failed to adequately understand or appropriately value the role of health as a key component of sustainable human development. It also realized that phenomena such as continued population increase, insecurity, civil strife, and the demographic shift toward higher numbers of elderly people all have major implications for our understanding of the determinants of health and the ways these factors contribute to health gains.

At the health level, the Commission recognized that disparities in health persist and grow across and within countries, an observation that pertains to both industrialized and developing countries. It also described the rapidly changing health context, including the health-transition phenomenon, with its "double burden of disease"; impacts of the economic crisis of the 1980s on the health status of populations; the increasing demand for curative services; the rising cost of care, reflecting the introduction of new technologies; and the range of new and different health actions.

At the health-research level, it felt that decision-makers and communities alike failed to assign an appropriate value to research, seeing it as peripheral to their interests and livelihoods. Particularly in developing countries (and also to some extent in industrialized countries), health research was largely unrelated to local concerns and realities; and the results of the research were frequently unavailable, or if they were available no one used them for policy or action. Box 1.1 reproduces the major findings of the Commission's report. Together they capture most of the concerns and descriptions of the problem found in other documents published at that time. However, the core finding of the Commission was that the international health-research system demonstrated "a gross mismatch between the burden of illness, which is overwhelmingly in the Third World, and investment in health research, which is overwhelmingly focused on the health problems of the industrialized countries" (CHRD 1990, p. xvii).

> **Box 1.1**
>
> **Major findings of the Commission on Health Research for Development**
>
> 1. The worldwide flow of resources supporting research on health problems of developing countries is very limited, and its application leaves large gaps. Greater amounts and more efficient application of resources are needed to support a major expansion and improvement of research activities and capacity within developing countries.
>
> 2. The enormous diversity of health circumstances speaks to the importance of priority setting at the national and international levels. Several major health problems are receiving attention; others appear relatively neglected. Major gaps exist with regard to information, monitoring, and assessment of the evolving health picture. Greater coherence of research responses to high-priority problems at the national and international levels is needed.
>
> 3. Developing-country scientists and institutions are pursuing a wide range of research activities, but greater productivity will require overcoming serious constraints — professional, institutional, and environmental. National commitment and international reinforcement for health research, specific actions to tackle constraints, and capacity building and maintenance within developing countries will all be necessary.
>
> 4. Appropriate contributions from industrialized countries should be expanded, focusing on advanced training, research, technical interaction, and participation in international partnership agreements. Rather than a system of new independent international centers, the major emphasis should be given to strengthening national centers and achieving "critical mass" and shared objectives through international networks of national centers.
>
> 5. The number and type of international research promotion programs are growing. These constitute the beginnings of a worldwide health research system. Joint efforts by United Nations agencies are noteworthy, and privately sponsored efforts have been productive. Stronger overall coherence is needed to reduce the fragmentation and competition induced by multiple, narrowly focused research initiatives.
>
> 6. Far too little attention is being given to the critical importance of building and sustaining individual and institutional health research capacity within developing countries. To remedy this problem leadership and commitment by national governments as well as longer-term support by international agencies will be necessary.
>
> Source: CHRD (1990, pp. 84–85).

THE COMMISSION AND WHAT HAPPENED NEXT

The idea of an independent commission on health research was a topic of discussion as early as 1985.[1] The justification for establishing a commission stemmed from three commonly held beliefs: developing countries had important unmet health needs; international health R&D activities could be more effective in meeting these needs; and donors were often unaware of promising opportunities to do so. Forty-seven individuals from around the world attended a planning meeting in Celigny, Switzerland, in July 1987, to clarify the problems and make recommendations on the desirability and nature of an independent international commission (Commission Secretariat 1987). The 16 sponsoring agencies selected a 12-person panel of three women and nine men (a remarkable range of eminent individuals, only four of whom were from industrialized countries). The work of the Commission was supported by a secretariat at Harvard University, with branches in London and Tokyo.

Why was this an "independent" Commission? The notes from the Celigny meeting describe a vigorous debate on whether the United Nations agencies should be sponsors. The United Nations Development Programme (UNDP) was already directly involved both in the discussion and eventually in the financial support of the Commission. But the attitude of many participants toward WHO was described as "ambiguous." Some believed that WHO would not welcome recommendations about health research from an "outside group." In fact, some commissioners described an ongoing tension between the Commission and WHO during the Commission's entire 2-year study. For example, WHO resisted the idea of distributing the Commission's report at the 1990 World Health Assembly. As well, the United Nations Children's Fund clearly advocated equity-oriented initiatives but was reluctant to invest directly in research. As it turned out, UNDP was the only United Nations agency listed as a Commission sponsor, although the World Bank provided some funds as well.

The Commission began its task in late 1987, using several strategies, such as full-Commission meetings (eight of these meetings over a period of 27 months, held in various parts of the world), collaborative workshops, secretariat workshops, and a range of consultative activities. In particular, developing-country leaders strongly participated through in-country collaborative workshops. Many working papers were submitted in the form of both country reports and contributed papers. More than 600 individuals helped to the formulate

---

[1] An account of these discussions, written by Joseph Cook of the Edna McConnell Clark Foundation, can be found as an annex of the report of the planning meeting, held in Celigny, Switzerland, 15–17 July 1987.

the Commission's vision of "a pluralistic worldwide health research system that will nurture productive national scientific groups linked together in transnational networks to address both national and global health problems" (CHRD 1990, p. xviii). The acknowledgments section of the report lists these individuals.

The Commission presented its report, *Health Research: Essential Link to Equity in Development* (CHRD 1990), at an international conference sponsored by the Nobel Assembly and supported by SAREC. The conference took place at the Karolinska Institute in Stockholm on 21–23 February 1990. Its objectives were threefold: to obtain an independent view of the Commission's work (about four-fifths of the 83 participants had not previously worked directly with the Commission), to define some next steps, and to identify issues for further elaboration. David Bradley, the conference rapporteur, stated in his report that the conference participants gave "extremely strong endorsement" to the four main recommendations of the Commission, as listed in the "Summary," above. A detailed presentation of the specific recommendations of the Commission's report is found in Box 1.2. These recommendations reflect the key messages of the Commission: that research can, in fact, contribute to the enhanced health and well-being of people in developing countries, that a major focus must be on building sustainable capacity at the country level, and that coalitions of research producers and users should address priority research problems.

Box 1.2

Specific recommendations of the Commission on Health Research for Development

Essential National Health Research

1. Developing countries should make careful plans for and carry out sustained, long-term programs for building research capacity and conducting ENHR [Essential National Health Research].

2. In doing so, each developing country should seek to (a) identify country-specific health problems and design and evaluate action programs for dealing with them, and (b) join in the international effort to find new knowledge, methods, and technologies for addressing global health problems that are of high priority for the country in question.

3. To build research capacity for ENHR, each developing country will need:
   — To invest in long-term development of the research capacity of individuals and institutions, especially in the fields of epidemiology, the social and policy sciences and management research;

(continued)

Box 1.2 continued.

- To set national priorities for research, for using both domestic and external resources;
- To accord professional recognition of good research and build career paths to attract and retain able researchers;
- To develop reliable and continuing links between researchers and research users; and
- To invest at least 2 percent of national health expenditures in ENHR.

International partnerships

1. Developing and industrialized countries and international agencies should promote the growth of collaborative international research networks as the principal means for mobilizing scientific talent to attack common problems.

2. Recognizing that research priorities will change over time, the Commission recommends:
   - Expanded support for existing and successful TDR [Special Programme for Research and Training in Tropical Diseases] and HRP [Special Programme of Research, Development and Research Training in Human Reproduction] programs;
   - Expanded support for two diarrheal disease programs, CDD [Programme for Control of Diarrhoeal Disease] and ICDDR,B [International Centre for Diarrheal Disease Research, Bangladesh];
   - Rapid expansion of research on acute respiratory infections, with special emphasis on simple and effective treatment;
   - Establishment of a research and action program on improved methods for case detection, ambulatory treatment, and prevention of tuberculosis;
   - Research in support of national programs to eradicate micronutrient deficiencies, especially of vitamin A, iron, and iodine;
   - Collaborative international research to identify modifiable factors to avert the high risk of diabetes, coronary heart disease, and hypertension associated with the health transition;
   - Design and assessment of behavioural interventions to reduce injuries, sexually transmitted diseases, and the growing threat of substance abuse;
   - Significant expansion of international collaborative research on mental health problems, emphasizing methods to diagnose and deal with the most prevalent and treatable conditions; and
   - Establishment of sustained international research networks in the areas of environmental and occupational health.

3. An international support system is needed to help developing countries strengthen country-specific health research capacity and action. It is recommended that:
   - The several international programs (HSR [health-systems research], Health Economics, INCLEN [International Clinical Epidemiology Network], and IHPP [International Health Policy Program] among others)

(continued)

Box 1.2 continued.

   that deal with selected aspects of country-specific health research be strengthened and coordinate their efforts at country level;
   — A facilitation unit to strengthen country-specific research be established to help developing countries achieve more efficient and effective national capacity building and to coordinate external linkages; the entity should be sponsored and supported by developing countries, United Nations agencies, bilateral donors, foundations, and other interested parties;
   — An annual meeting of scientists, health leaders, and donor representatives interested in country-specific health research be sponsored by developing countries, development agencies, and foundations to promote information exchange about research results and methods and to mobilize financial and technical assistance;
   — International awards for distinguished contributions to country-specific health research be established and presented each year at the annual country-specific health research meeting to three to five young leaders in this field of research.

4. As a major resource for addressing health problems of developing countries, industrialized-country health research and training institutions should:
   — Provide career opportunities for young scientists to become engaged in research on health problems of developing countries;
   — Promote the strengthening of schools of public health, tropical disease institutes, medical schools, and development studies groups to pursue advanced research, conduct training, and participate in international networks;
   — Commit a larger share of the budgets of health research funding agencies to support research focused on the health problems of developing countries.

5. WHO [World Health Organization], UNDP [United Nations Development Programme], the development banks, and other agencies should strengthen or augment existing international research-promotion programs, increase their own investments in health research and research capacity strengthening, and reinvigorate research review bodies.

Mobilizing research funding

1. Developing countries, bilateral and multilateral development agencies, industrialized-country research agencies, foundations, NGOs [non-governmental organizations], and the pharmaceutical industry should all raise funding levels for health research. Specifically:
   — Developing countries should invest at least 2 percent of national health expenditures in research and research capacity strengthening, and
   — At least 5 percent of project and program aid for the health sector from development aid agencies should be earmarked for research and research capacity strengthening.

(continued)

> **Box 1.2 concluded.**
>
> 2. The quality of research and research strengthening efforts, as well as their quantity, needs improvement. Specifically:
>   — Much longer time horizons should be used for research capacity building than has been customary in the past;
>   — Innovative financing strategies such as debt-for-health-research swaps, funding pools, and funding intermediaries should be explored; and
>   — Foundations and special research agencies such as IDRC [International Development Research Centre] and SAREC [Swedish Agency for Research Cooperation with Developing Countries] should continue their pioneering roles in addressing new needs in innovative ways and in mobilizing broader support for major research programs.
>
> **Forum for Review and Advocacy**
>
> An international mechanism should be established to monitor progress in health research and, when needed, to promote financial and technical support for research on health problems of the developing world. The mechanism should be sufficiently independent to be objective in its recommendations, and therefore its mandate should not be to operate research programs but to promote action by others.
>
> Source: CHRD (1990, pp. 88–89).

The Stockholm conference (later referred to as the First International Conference on Health Research for Development) included presentations from five countries already engaged in ENHR activities: Indonesia, Mexico, Philippines, Thailand, and Zimbabwe. Concerning the way ahead, the conference participants agreed unanimously on two parallel activities: to immediately "assist committed countries to maintain the momentum of ENHR and to build research capacity, and encourage others to join in" (SAREC 1990, p. 31); and to make an ongoing international effort "to advocate and sustain ENHR, to mobilize resources and to facilitate networks of support, interaction and collaboration in research" (SAREC 1990, p. 31). Specifically, the conference recommended the creation of an interim task force to function for 2 years to allow time to establish longer term mechanisms (a secretariat and a council). The final sentence in the conference report urged leaders from developing countries "to take the key role in moving ahead the recommendations of the Report" (SAREC 1990, p. 36). (In Box 1.3, two former Commission members reflect on the major impacts of the Commission and its 1990 report.)

> **Box 1.3**
>
> ### Impact of the independent Commission on Health Research for Development and its 1990 report
>
> Former Commission Chair, Dr John Evans, and Commission member Dr Adetokunbo Lucas, recently spoke with COHRED (COHRED Newsletter 2000) about what they perceived to be the major impacts of the Commission and its 1990 report, *Health Research: Essential Link to Equity in Development* (CHRD 1990).
>
> **Dr John Evans**
> The central conclusion of the Commission was that every country needed an analytic capability rooted in measurement and social sciences, as well as biomedical science, to inform its decisions on the use of limited resources to meet the health needs of its population. The Commission focused attention on the needs, or demand side, of health policy and programs and the importance of local circumstances in the successful implementation of health programs. The enormous investment in health research in the industrialized world had achieved an avalanche of biomedical and technological advances but little served the predominant health needs of three-quarters of the world's population living in developing countries.
> The Commission made the case not only for strengthening local health-research capability in Third World countries but also for broadening the relevant sciences, particularly the measurement and social sciences, as important components of institutional strengthening. As well, it drew attention to the fact that translation of evidence into policy was an active, skill-demanding process and not something that flowed spontaneously from the power of the evidence. More broadly, the Commission stressed that research was not merely an academic exercise outside the mainstream objectives of health organizations but an essential and integral component of their strategy to meet health needs and to manage health programs (COHRED Newsletter 1999).
>
> **Dr Adetokunbo Lucas**
> One of the major impacts I saw from the Commission report was that it awakened interest in the need for research at the country level. This — tied in with the idea that we must not undertake health research solely for the sake of research as such but in order to promote health and equity in health — was the first time I had seen research being actively promoted as the key to equity in health and development. It was successful in establishing a number of targets, which at the very least provided us with benchmarks with which to measure progress toward attaining equity in health.

In May 1990, shortly after the Stockholm conference, the Technical Discussions of the 43rd World Health Assembly in Geneva focused on the role of health research in the strategy for Health for All by the Year 2000 (HFA/2000). At this meeting, the Commission first distributed its report, despite initial WHO resistance. Participants at this meeting agreed that health research should become an integral component of national strategies for achieving HFA/2000. The Assembly's resolution (43.19) on the Role of Health Research included a call to all member states to undertake essential health research appropriate to their national needs (Davies and Mansourian 1992). Much of the wording in the resolution reinforced the recommendations of the Commission.

Before the end of the year (November 1990), an international conference on ENHR took place in Pattaya, Thailand. At this conference, participants from developing countries identified seven elements in the implementation of ENHR: promotion and advocacy, ENHR mechanism, priority-setting, capacity-building and capacity-strengthening, networking, financing, and evaluation. The Task Force later disseminated these in a 1991 publication, *Essential National Health Research: A Strategy for Action in Health and Human Development* (TFHRD 1991), which included descriptions of the ENHR process in Mexico, Mozambique, Philippines, and Thailand.

As mandated by the Stockholm conference, IDRC and SAREC collaborated to establish the Task Force. Its several members had also been members of the Commission, including Professor V. Ramalingaswami of India, who served as Task Force chair. A secretariat based in the UNDP offices in Geneva supported the Task Force. Its original plan was to work in depth with a small number of countries. But interest in the ENHR process was intense, and over a 2-year period the Task Force was working with more than 20 countries. These countries saw ENHR as a powerful and innovative strategy to plan, prioritize, and manage national health research and mobilize its three main constituencies: researchers, policymakers, and the community.

Following a pattern begun by the Commission, the IDRC office in New Delhi published and distributed a monthly newsletter (*ENHR Forum*). Working groups were formed, including one with the task of recommending longer term mechanisms to support ENHR. Another working group focused on monitoring progress.

These working groups consulted widely with many stakeholders, including WHO. The work of the Task Force culminated in the Second International Conference on Health Research for Development, held in Geneva in March 1993 (COHRED 1993). (Box 1.4 gives a list of key events in health R&D over the past 15 years.)

At this conference, representatives from 18 countries (as well as Commonwealth Caribbean countries as a group) presented their experiences with ENHR. The proceedings of this conference describe

> **Box 1.4**
>
> **Health research for development: key events**
>
> 1986 WHO ACHR report: *Health research strategy*
>
> 1987 Celigny meeting (pre-Commission)
> First meeting of the Commission
>
> 1990 Commission report presented in Stockholm
> 43rd World Health Assembly: "The Role of Health Research in the Strategy for Health for All by the Year 2000"
> International Conference on ENHR: Pattaya, Thailand
>
> 1991 Task Force on Health Research for Development begins its work
>
> 1993 Council on Health Research for Development (COHRED) created
> World Bank publishes *World development report 1993: investing in health*
> Ottawa conference: Future partnership for the acceleration of health development
>
> 1996 Ad Hoc Committee publishes *Investing in health research and development*
> COHRED interim assessment
>
> 1997 WHO ACHR report: *A research policy agenda for science and technology to support global health development*
> Global Forum for Health Research #1
> World Bank publication: *Sector strategy: health, nutrition, and population*
>
> 1998 Global Forum #2
>
> 1999 Global Forum #3
> WHO creates Department of Research Policy & Cooperation
>
> 2000 International Conference on Health Research for Development, Bangkok

an extensive debate on an ongoing mechanism to facilitate and coordinate ENHR. Eventually, conference participants adopted a Declaration of Health Research for Development, supporting a mechanism called the Council on Health Research for Development (or COHRED). This was a direct response to one of the recommendations of the Commission on supporting country initiatives. Immediately after the conference, on 10 March 1993, the Constituting Assembly formally adopted statutes and implementing regulations, and COHRED was born. By the end of June, it had a 17-member Board and was registered as an NGO in Switzerland (although COHRED retained its formal links with UNDP). Meanwhile, five countries had completed their ENHR plans and were ready to present them to prospective partners.

Over the years, COHRED has continued to assist a steadily increasing number of countries in exploring and implementing ENHR. In Africa, Asia, and the Commonwealth Caribbean, it has created regional ENHR networks to facilitate work at the national level. In addition, a variety of both regional and global working groups and projects have captured the experience of the ENHR strategy and built further capacities for it. Using several communication strategies (such as a quarterly newsletter, a website, and a range of publications), COHRED has attempted to capture the experiences of ENHR and thus contribute to a growing knowledge base on this approach. It has also made efforts in capacity development for ENHR, often through partnerships with other like-minded networks and organizations. (Chapter 8 gives a description of COHRED activities.)

On the eve of the next international conference on health research for development, COHRED is also playing an important role as one of several partner organizations reviewing the experience of health research for development over the past 10 years and devising a global strategy for the first years of the new millennium.

HEALTH RESEARCH IN THE 1990S: THE ROLES AND ACTIVITIES OF WHO, GFHR, THE WORLD BANK, AND OTHER INTERNATIONAL PROGRAMS

THE WORLD HEALTH ORGANIZATION

As the principal NGO for health, WHO has traditionally seen its role as one of having a "wider vision and larger responsibility" than other institutions and organizations engaged in health research. As articulated in the 1986 report of the WHO Advisory Committee on Health Research, WHO is able to view health problems from a historical and global perspective and, as a result, "assess the determinants of health, and arrive at a just balance between preventive and therapeutic measures, between basic and applied research and between the needs of developed and developing countries" (ACHR 1986, p. 43). Although WHO itself is not primarily a research organization, it facilitates and supports research in collaboration with other agencies, through programs such as the long-running Special Programme of Research, Development and Research Training in Human Reproduction and the Special Programme for Research and Training in Tropical Diseases (TDR). WHO also incorporates its research into its regular programs, such as those on diarrheal diseases and essential drugs. Its various technical programs and their expert committees have responsibility for developing and monitoring its research strategy. Global and regional Advisory Committees on Health Research (ACHRs) provide broad guidelines.

Throughout the latter part of the 1980s and into the 1990s, WHO's goal of achieving HFA/2000 has shaped its research strategy. In 1984, WHO's director general requested its ACHR (then titled the Advisory Committee on Medical Research [ACMR]) to outline a fresh health-research strategy in light of HFA/2000. Chaired by Professor T. McKeown, a specially appointed subcommittee of ACMR recommended that WHO promote research in five priority areas to "raise the health of all people to an acceptable level as rapidly as possible" (ACHR 1986, p. 22). ACMR recommended that WHO's first priority should be to encourage research on diseases of poverty and the tropics. Other recommended priorities included diseases of affluence (that is, noncommunicable illnesses predominant in developed countries and threatening to advance into developing countries), treatment and care of the sick, and delivery of health services. ACMR also resolved that WHO should strive to improve the quality of research so that certain minimum standards would be maintained throughout the world and should continue to support research trainees from developing countries.

WHO revisited its role in health research 6 years later, in May 1990, during the Technical Discussions of the 43rd World Health Assembly (where the Commission first distributed its report). These technical discussions focused on health-systems research, research capacity-strengthening, nutrition, and advances in science and technology (S&T). The Assembly called on WHO to take on a more active leadership role in monitoring disease patterns, advances in research, and resource flows; informing a global research agenda; coordinating the health-research policies of various international players; and promoting selected directions in health research, particularly national health-systems research (HSR) and nutrition. It requested the director general to work in collaboration with the global and regional ACHRs and "use appropriate mechanisms to assess new and emerging areas of science and technology, investigate evolving problems of critical significance to health and identify appropriate methodologies for trend assessment and forecasting, including epidemiology" (Davies and Mansourian 1992, p. 209). Such monitoring would position WHO "to promote the harmonization of science and research policies in health between the WHO, the UN system and other international agencies and organizations" (Davies and Mansourian 1992, p. 209). In addition, it encouraged WHO to strengthen its capacity to support countries developing HSR and set an example by incorporating it into its own action programs. Similarly, it urged WHO to give nutrition a higher research profile so that member states would follow suit.

WHO was a full partner with the World Bank in preparing the *World Development Report 1993: Investing in Health* (World Bank 1993) (see below). In particular, WHO contributed to a jointly sponsored assessment of the global burden of disease, a major feature of the report. Shortly after its release, IDRC hosted a "next-steps" international conference in Ottawa (IDRC 1993). IDRC, WHO, and the World Bank cosponsored the conference, which had three major outcomes:

— WHO would serve as the secretariat for an ad hoc review of health-research priorities (see below);

— With support from the Canadian government, IDRC would initiate a research project to test the development of nationally defined health-intervention packages, health-policy reform, and improved donor coordination (as recommended in the *World Development Report 1993*) (this became the Tanzania Essential Health Intervention Project); and

— The World Bank would lead an initiative to examine issues in increasing and redirecting investment into equity-oriented health development.

Three years later, WHO published the 1996 report of its Ad Hoc Committee on Health Research Relating to Future Intervention Options, entitled *Investing in Health Research and Development* (Ad Hoc Committee 1996). The Ad Hoc Committee convened under the auspices of WHO at the request of a number of health-research investors, including governments, bilateral and multilateral development-assistance agencies, and private foundations present at the 1993 Ottawa conference. It reviewed the health needs and related priorities for R&D in low- to middle-income countries. The intention of its report was "to contribute to an agenda for international action in which individual nations' agendas inform global priorities and global needs and experience influence national agendas" (Ad Hoc Committee 1996, p. xxi). The issues of resource allocation and efficiency, which crept into the 1990 Technical Discussions in terms of "doing the most with less," were the focus of the 1996 Ad Hoc Committee report. It argued for the need to make "hard choices" to direct limited resources to areas of greatest need and promise.

The Ad Hoc Committee outlined a systematic approach to allocating health-research funds. Its five-step strategy included calculating the burden of disease, identifying reasons for the persistence of the burden, judging the adequacy of the current knowledge base, assessing the promise of the R&D effort (with special attention to cost-effectiveness), and determining how much is already being done about the problem. The result was a list of "best buys," or key investments, along with some other initiatives applied to four "unfinished agenda" health challenges: maternal and child health, continually changing microbial threats, noncommunicable illnesses and injuries, and health policy and systems.

Among these best buys were three new proposed initiatives: Research and Training on Non-communicable Diseases and Healthy Aging; Research, Training and Capacity-Building on Injuries; and Research and Training on Health Systems and Policy — along with a mechanism to review global health needs, assess R&D opportunities, and monitor resource flows. The proposed mechanism would take advice from scientific advisory groups already involved in enabling health research at national and international levels, such as the WHO global and regional ACHRs, scientific and advisory groups of existing international research programs, and organizations such as COHRED, INCLEN, and IHPP. The mechanism (which would become known as GFHR) would then present its recommendations and conclusions to existing programs for implementation.

The tenor of the Ad Hoc Committee's report demonstrates that by the mid-1990s the problem confronting the international health R&D community had been reframed to include not just the gross imbalances in burden of illness, investment in health research, and research capacity within and between countries, but the fragmented nature of the community itself and the resulting inefficiencies and lack of coordination of effort and resources. In short,

> the distribution of resources and effort across the spectrum of health problems [is seen] to reflect uneven advocacy and special pleading rather than rational and coordinated responses to need. Some work is duplicated, significant gaps remain, and the dispersion of resources constrains capacity to focus resources on high-priority problems.
> — Ad Hoc Committee (1996, p. xxxiv)

The challenge of creating a pluralistic, worldwide health-research system as envisioned by the Commission (in which the various partners exchange information, link their efforts, and base resource-allocation decisions on explicit analysis of priorities) was taken up on two fronts: by WHO's ACHR and by the newly initiated GFHR. In 1997,

ACHR published *A Research Policy Agenda for Science and Technology to Support Global Health Development* (ACHR 1997). The research-policy agenda highlighted a number "domain-based" global "research imperatives and opportunities," indicating the scope and variety of needed research, as opposed to a ranked list of disease-based global research priorities.[2] The research agenda outlined a strategy to "initiate and sustain a systematic, dynamic process of dialogue, joint planning and multidisciplinary participation in research" (ACHR 1997, p. 36). WHO would exploit modern information and communication technologies to create a global planning network for health research, comprising "intelligent" research networks built on common themes and critical issues.[3] To initiate the development work for such a global planning network, ACHR has, on behalf of WHO, sponsored the Planet HERES (Planning Network for Health Research) project.

In 1998, WHO appointed Dr Gro Brundtland its new director general. Within a few months, WHO undertook a major restructuring at its Geneva-based headquarters, including a reconsideration of internal mechanisms to support WHO's R&D. WHO commissioned an internal working group in late 1998, along with an external Board of Advisors. The working group recommended that WHO create a Department of Research Policy and Cooperation within the cluster of Evidence and Information for Policy, and this new department started operations in August 1999. It has the following objective (WHO 2000[4]):

> to stimulate research for, with and by developing countries through:
> — The ability to identify emerging trends in scientific knowledge with the potential to improve health;
> — The mobilization of the world research community toward tackling priority health problems;
> — The development of initiatives aimed at strengthening research capacity in the developing world with the ultimate aim of enshrining research as a foundation for policy.

---

[2] The ACHR Health Profile posits five domains of determinants of global health: environment, food and nutrition, sociocultural factors, health-care systems, and disease conditions and health impairments.

[3] "Intelligent" refers to "the characteristic achieved by linking, through networking and communication technologies and knowledge-based technical know-how of researchers for the purpose of solving specific research problems using the minimal pathway approach" (ACHR 1997, p. 41).

[4] WHO (World Health Organization). 2000. Strategic plan: Department of Research Policy and Cooperation, 20 Mar. Unpublished memo.

THE GLOBAL FORUM FOR HEALTH RESEARCH

The Ad Hoc Committee presented its findings in Geneva in June 1996, at a meeting of researchers, government officials, and representatives of NGOs and donor agencies. The participants endorsed the Ad Hoc Committee's findings, particularly the creation of a mechanism to review global health needs, assess R&D opportunities, and monitor resource flows. One year later, in June 1997, GFHR began its work. Its functions have included providing a forum for stakeholders to review global health-research priorities, promoting ongoing analysis of the global health-research situation (including resource flows), and facilitating coalition-building for research on important global problems. GFHR has thus become part of the Commission's recommended international mechanism to monitor and convene discussion on global themes, allowing COHRED to work directly with countries to facilitate the ENHR strategy (see Box 1.2).

GFHR is an independent entity and is registered as a Swiss foundation. It is managed by a council of 20 members representing government policymakers, multilateral and bilateral development agencies, foundations, international NGOs, women's associations, research institutions, and the private sector. The GFHR Secretariat, located at the WHO headquarters in Geneva, started its operations in January 1998.

GFHR's mandate is to work to correct the alarming disparity in worldwide health-research expenditures (widely referred to as the "10/90 disequilibrium"). This disparity concerns an estimated 56 billion United States dollars (USD) a year, of which 90% is spent on research on health problems that concern only 10% of the world's population. GFHR selected five strategies to achieve its goal: organize an annual forum, undertake analytical work in priority-setting, promote partnership initiatives in priority health-research areas, disseminate information about the 10/90 disequilibrium, and evaluate and monitor progress in correcting this gap.

Among the outputs of GFHR is "a practical framework for setting priorities in health research," published in *The 10/90 Report on Health Research 1999* (GFHR 1999). This framework relies on the five-step process outlined by the Ad Hoc Committee in 1996. It uses the Visual Health Information Profile, advanced in the research-policy agenda of WHO's ACHR, to assess priority research areas at the local, national, regional, or global level. It has also been a supporting partner in a series of concerted initiatives to address key health problems. These initiatives include the WHO-led Global Tuberculosis Research Initiative, Initiative on Control of Cardiovascular Diseases in Developing

Countries, MIM, International AIDS Vaccine Initiative (IAVI), and the Alliance for Health Services and Health Systems Research. A special program called the Public/Private Partnerships Initiative addresses the inaccessibility of drugs and vaccines for the poor. GFHR has created a secretariat to assess these partnerships and facilitate new ones, such as the recent Medicines for Malaria Venture (GFHR 2000).

THE WORLD BANK

As a primarily financial institution, the World Bank jointly supports or finances health-research programs or initiatives, such as TDR, MIM, and IAVI. Its internal research activities focus on economic policy as applied to the health, nutrition, and population (HNP) sector. Although focused on health systems rather than health research, the *World Development Report 1993* (World Bank 1993) had a significant impact on discussions in this sector. It reiterated the Commission's recommendation to establish a global mechanism for better coordination of international health research. It also made a case for allocating resources for epidemiological and health-policy research to increase evidence-based decision-making, as well as research on national research priorities. Of equal importance was its emphasis on misallocation and waste (in addition to inequities) in world health spending. One of its key messages concerned the need to reduce inefficiencies and improve cost-effectiveness, a message that has broadened the formulation of problems confronting the international health R&D community.

Since the publication of this significant report the World Bank has steadily increased its investment in health-sector reform. Representatives of the World Bank's health group have been actively involved in many of the discussions and initiatives in health research for development. The Bank has also become a significant source of health-research funding. For example, the 1997 *Sector Strategy: Health, Nutrition and Population* stated that

> *country-specific research and analysis of HNP (Health, Nutrition and Population) issues supported through Bank loans and credits has* [sic] *recently ranged between approximately US$50 and US$75 million per year. This is 5 to 6 percent of total lending and by far the largest source of external research funding for HNP in client countries.*
> — World Bank Group (1997, p. 11)

In addition, the World Bank's Policy Research Department has spent more than 1 million USD annually on HNP issues.

OTHER INTERNATIONAL PROGRAMS

Over the past 10–15 years, a number of international programs (in addition to those linked to WHO) were created to build health-research capacity in developing countries. They have been important contributors to all aspects of health research for development over this period. For example, in early 1990, when the Commission was about to release its report, a group of nine international programs issued a joint statement, the Puebla Declaration. It supported the main thrust of the Commission's recommendations, particularly on capacity development (see TFHRD 1991). Each of these programs has undergone its own distinctive evolution during this period. Brief summaries of some of these programs appear below.

International Clinical Epidemiology Network

INCLEN began work in 1982, as a result of the leadership of Dr Kerr White, who was concerned about the continuing "schism" between public health and clinical medicine. White's vision was to train established clinicians from developing-country universities in the science of public health and epidemiology. Supported largely by the Rockefeller Foundation, INCLEN has prepared about 300 individuals in 30 countries to conduct priority-driven research and teach health-research methods. Beginning with four training centres in Australia, Canada, and the United States, INCLEN has evolved to the point of having centres in developing countries take over the training function. In the last 2 years, INCLEN's priorities have shifted from capacity development to multicountry health research on specific issues, and INCLEN has evolved into a more regional structure.

International Health Policy Program

Initiated in 1986, with the support of the Pew Charitable Trusts (and later the Carnegie Corporation and the World Bank), IHPP has been concerned about resource issues in effective, equity-oriented health policies. Its principle activity has been to provide support for groups engaged in health-policy analysis and development in Africa and Asia, and it has also awarded Career Development Fellowships, sponsored participants' meetings and authors' workshops, and disseminated policy-related research findings.

Applied Research on Child Health project

The ARCH project succeeds the Applied Diarrheal Disease Research project, which supported 150 research studies in 16 countries. Based in the Harvard Institute for International Development and funded largely through the United States Agency for International Development, the ARCH project focuses on the principal causes of infant and child morbidity and mortality. ARCH supports applied research in developing countries through research grants and technical assistance to groups of social and health scientists.

The Multilateral Initiative on Malaria

The more recent initiative, MIM, grew out of an awareness of fragmentation in malaria research, with various organizations independently supporting separate research projects. A January 1997 meeting in Dakar, Senegal, to focus on the malaria problem in Africa identified broad research priorities and needs. Shortly after this, MIM invited the Wellcome Trust in London to serve as the coordinating secretariat for its activities, which now involve advocacy (including fund-raising), facilitation in the areas of coordination and collaboration, and information exchange. An example of its efforts is the Malaria Research and Reference Reagent Repository in Dakar. It has convened major conferences in Durban (in 1999) and Abuja (in 2000). In collaboration with TDR, MIM has created a special task force on Malaria Research Capability Strengthening in Africa. With a commitment to working closely with WHO's Roll Back Malaria project, MIM is helping to ensure links between research and control activities. The various organizations involved have appeared to welcome MIM, and it is helping to synergize the efforts of researchers, funders, and others committed to addressing this important regional problem.

Special industrialized-country initiatives

Over the past two decades or more, a number of industrialized countries have undertaken special initiatives to support research in developing countries. A few examples are described below.

Sweden — Stimulated by the inclusion of a global action program for S&T in the United Nations Second Development Decade (the 1970s), the Swedish parliament commissioned an inquiry into the organization of research on problems in developing countries. A report, *Research for Development*, was published in 1973. This report articulated (among other recommendations) some guiding principles for development research: problem orientation, multi- or interdisciplinarity, value (or development relevance), and focus on the developing countries. With these principles as a foundational framework, Sweden created SAREC in 1975. Its major task is to contribute to building research capacity in some of the world's poorest countries, through support for universities. In the health sector, this policy has resulted in long-term support for health research at universities in such countries as Ethiopia, Mozambique, and Tanzania. SAREC has also supported direct cooperation between institutions in developing countries and Sweden.

By the mid-1990s, SAREC had 380 joint projects involving more than 100 Swedish university departments. At the time of its incorporation into the larger Swedish International Development Agency, in the mid-1990s, SAREC reevaluated its long-term support for research capacity development. It recognized that it needed to take supportive measures for the university as a whole as a supplement to research cooperation, such as through broad support for higher education, research, and university administration. Overall, this 25-year experience of supporting development research has been worth the investment.

Canada — Canada has stimulated and supported development research through IDRC, an autonomous public corporation established in 1970 through an Act of the Canadian parliament. It was the first development-assistance institution to focus exclusively on research for the development of S&T. During the 1970s and 1980s, it implemented its programs through such sectors as agriculture and health. In 1988, through its Health Sciences Division, IDRC was a major supporter of the Commission. During the late 1980s and early 1990s, it adopted a new strategy — empowerment through knowledge — emphasizing the central importance of research capacity development. In 1992, the United Nations Conference on Environment and Development in Rio de Janeiro gave IDRC an expanded mandate to represent (through a revised program framework) Canada's major contribution to Agenda 21. In 1995, as a consequence of reductions in the federal budget, IDRC downsized its operations and replaced its four division structures with six program themes.

It revealed a new corporate framework in 1997, reflecting lessons learned in 25 years of "success, failure, and persistence" (IDRC 1997, p. 7). It identified three lessons: societies build their own future; knowledge is the key (and information is no longer a substitute for knowledge); and single approaches do not yield results (complex problems require multidisciplinary approaches). For example, a current IDRC research initiative is Macroeconomic Adjustment Policies, Health Sector Reform, and Health Care in the South. More recently, IDRC has provided leadership to coordinate research on the global health problem caused by tobacco.

Switzerland — In 1994, SCRPDC was established under the auspices of the Conference of the Swiss Academies of Science. SCRPDC's mandate is to define and promote a "Swiss strategy for the Promotion of Research in Development Countries" (SCRPDC 1998, p. 3) and to encourage Swiss scientists to participate in this endeavour. An example of the work of this commission is its recent *Guidelines for Research in Partnership with Developing Countries* (SCRPDC 1998), which describes 11 principles of research partnership (see Box 6.3).

CONCLUDING REMARKS

Over the past 10–15 years, awareness and analysis of the disequilibrium problem in health research for development have clearly increased, and this has been matched to some extent by increased action. Now there are organizations like COHRED (working directly with developing countries) and GFHR (providing a global venue for monitoring and discussion). These organizations were not in existence 10 years ago. Such organizations have identified health-research priorities at both national and global levels. And major organizations (WHO, for example), international programs, and countries (both developing and industrialized) have intensified their efforts to work in partnership with others to address these national and global health-research priorities.

However, the current "international mechanism" (to use a phrase from the Commission's recommendation) is still too fragmented, slow-moving, and uncoordinated. Moreover, the system's performance falls far short of its potential in monitoring progress, promoting financial and technical support for developing countries, and accelerating capacity development.

In contrast, an international institution in the global agricultural sector has been instrumental in "sowing the seeds of the green revolution" during these past 15 years (World Bank 1999, p. 4). This is the Consultative Group on International Agricultural Research (CGIAR). Created in 1971, its membership includes both developing and industrialized countries, as well as private foundations and international organizations such as the Food and Agriculture Organization of the United Nations. The key strategy has been to create and support 16 international research centres and train a great many scientists and technicians. According to the World Bank's *World Development Report 1989/99: Knowledge for Development* (World Bank 1999), CGIAR has made a major contribution to the development and use of new agricultural technologies. As a result, through increased yields in crops, the global production of food has kept up with a steadily increasing demand, in a world where "90 million new mouths must be fed every year" (World Bank 1999, p. 131). Over the past decade, CGIAR has expanded its scope to include research on environmental issues, forestry, aquatic resources, and the interrelationships of these factors with agricultural research. As a publicly funded global organization, it has also steadily increased its interaction with research institutions in the private sector. But it has not ensured strong national systems of agricultural research and production. And global food insecurity is still a problem for 790 million people. CGIAR recognizes the need to respond to a changing environment and is moving toward more "virtual" institutions and an increasing emphasis on impact assessment.

Can we truly say that over the past 10 years the global health-research community has contributed directly to a "health revolution," analogous to the green revolution? Given the realities of achieving change over a 10-year time span, where have we made definite contributions? Where have we fallen short? What have been the facilitating and impeding factors? Have the recommended investments been made and appropriately targeted? Why is cooperation among various organizations and institutions still perceived as inadequate?

Some of these questions are addressed in subsequent chapters of this book, primarily from the perspective of developing countries. Other issues will be addressed at the October 2000 international conference. The debate must lead us to respond boldly and creatively to the question of how to intensify our efforts in the next 10 years to ensure that health research contributes maximally as an essential link to equity in development.

CHAPTER 2

HEALTH FOR SOME: HEALTH, POVERTY, AND EQUITY AT THE BEGINNING OF THE 21ST CENTURY

Tessa Tan-Torres Edejer

SUMMARY

People agree that equity is of paramount importance in health and development. Beyond that, they are reluctant to explicitly conceptualize and commit to a realistic vision of equity in health. This is now the single most serious impediment to progress in addressing health inequities.

Societies must gain consensus on two pivotal issues:

— Equality of what (health, access, use, expenditures)?

— Equity among whom (income classes, gender, ethnic grouping, geography, religion)?

The policy dilemma, however, is in deciding how much inequality is inequitable. Responding realistically to this dilemma reflects what a society judges fair and what ill-health it judges avoidable.

Longevity accompanied by health for all is a common goal. Because of the nature of health, though, we cannot distribute it equally. At most, we can distribute a probability of attaining a good health outcome through an intervention. Narrowly interpreted, "equality" would mean equal access to or use of services. However, a broader interpretation would include considerations of both horizontal equity, which requires that people with the same needs receive the same services, and vertical equity, which requires that people with greater needs receive greater services. Amartya Sen (1992) argued for the goal of "equal capabilities," where society ensures that each individual has the capability of converting an opportunity to its full potential benefit. This broadens the concept of need to include more than a medical indication and broadens the concept of opportunity to include more than health care.

Equality is value free, whereas equity is normative. Saying something is unequal is to describe a phenomenon; however, ascribing the differentials to the systematic effect of a variable is potentially to transform the description into a judgment: if the variable is a social grouping considered unfair and the differential is thought significant and avoidable, then what is unequal is said to be inequitable.

When someone has no choice in his living or working conditions, then any resulting ill-health or lack of informed access to potential remedies can be judged unfair. What ill-health is judged avoidable is often affected by what is felt to be affordable or efficient in or outside the health sector. Consequently, some people regard the health of the rich as a benchmark of avoidable ill-health. Others would prefer setting a minimum acceptable level of health while defending the individual's right to purchase services over and above the minimum standard. Equity in health thus implies a society's commitment to individuals' being equally capable of achieving good health outcomes and is conditional on respecting the diversity and autonomy of these individuals and achieved through taking action for the health of unfairly disadvantaged people.

Despite the limitations of proxy data in measuring inequity, they project a compelling picture of the widespread prevalence of inequities in health. Reanalysis of the 1990 Global Burden of Disease data showed that communicable diseases cause 47.3% of deaths and 49.8% of disability-adjusted life years' (DALY) loss shouldered by the poorest 20% of the population, whereas the richest 20% bear only 4.2% of deaths and 2.6% of DALY loss caused by communicable disease. Other health indicators show differentials of 2- to 10-fold between rich and poor. Studies demonstrate health gradients across socioeconomic groupings even within developed countries, where the major causes of death are noncommunicable illnesses and the poorest quintile may in reality be the nearly or working poor.

The effects of poverty on the health of individuals can easily be ascribed to its social consequences in feelings of risk, powerlessness, vulnerability, and low self-esteem, as well as to the absolute effect of material deprivation. Empirical evidence shows that not only the incomes of individuals but also the distribution of their incomes within a society affects their health. Thus, in addition to the absolute impact of material deprivation, a socioeconomic gradient has an independent effect on health. Some have advanced the loss of social capital (the cohesion and solidarity of a society) as a plausible mechanism to explain many deleterious health effects.

Thus, new findings have generated enthusiasm for a social model of health that is based on the notions that

— The welfare of the community is as important as the health of the individual; and

— At the individual level, the interpersonal aspects of health care are as important as the technical ones.

The social model of health recognizes the value of creating opportunities for community action, building social capital, and infusing health care with a genuine concern for the individual's personhood and autonomy.

This shift from a biomedical to a social model of health permits a broadening of the equity goal to include substantive equity, achieved through acceptable equalization of the individual's capability of benefiting from health actions, with priority given to the disadvantaged. This broadening of the equity goal also permits inclusion of procedural equity, obtained to the extent that the structure, process, or procedures to achieve substantive equity are fair.

At the beginning of the 21st century, inequities in health are still prevalent. Yet, a number of studies have made considerable advances in the understanding of poverty and ill-health at the individual and community levels. The definition of poverty now includes the social consequences of risk, vulnerability, and powerlessness. We now link the health of the individual to that of the community, and this has allowed us to develop a social model of health and novel approaches to health action beyond biomedicine.

PUTTING EQUITY INTO A REAL-LIFE CONTEXT

Last year, an international newsweekly carried a report about a father who sold one of his kidneys to pay for the hospitalization of his child (who had severe measles), and thus a stranger received a life-saving kidney transplant (Baguioro 1999). This is a real-life tragedy about two people, each desperate to save his or her own life or the life of a loved one. Linked by forced choices, one becomes a buyer and the other a seller in the illicit trade in body parts. But this story has a subplot — a subplot about fairness and how people have divergent levels of access to knowledge and resources. One of these people could afford to purchase the high-technology care needed to prolong his or her life; the other had no resources, aside from his body, to parlay into a chance to prevent his child from dying prematurely. He probably did not know (or could not act on his knowledge) that measles could be effectively prevented using a widely available, single-shot vaccine. This is perhaps the most tragic element of the story.

Many versions of such stories occur in many parts of the world in real life.[1] Is this equitable? Should society be concerned? What does society owe to all of us in terms of our health? Are these just rhetorical questions?

DEFINING EQUITY IN HEALTH

The most serious impediment to progress in the field of equity in health is the lack of any explicit consensus on what constitutes equity or, perhaps more importantly, what constitutes **in**equity. Today, *equity* seems to be just one of the trendy words winning approval and instantaneous acceptance in politics. No one questions the importance of equity. As a result of the backlash from the single-minded focus on cost-cutting in the 1980s, coupled with a vague, ever-present fear of globalization, equity in health has become of paramount concern.

Equity is a normative term, and unlike *equality*, which is a value-free description of a distribution, equity implies judgment (see Box 2.1). Thus, society needs to agree on the conceptualization of equity. Although concepts of equity are not right or wrong, approaches to monitoring and ensuring progress toward equity can be consistent or inconsistent (Mooney 1994). Each society must obtain consensus on two key issues in the conceptualization of equity in health: **Equality of what** (health, access to health care, or use of health care)? and **Equity among whom** (socioeconomic class, gender, race, geography)? Invariably, obtaining a consensus on these two issues will require clarification of the philosophical framework and values upheld in each society.

In 1990, the Commission on Health Research for Development published its findings in *Health Research: Essential Link to Equity and Development* (CHRD 1990). In the introduction to the report, the Commission gave examples of health disparities among and within nations (industrialized versus developing, black versus white, poor versus middle income or affluent, rural versus urban), mainly in terms

---

[1] This chapter focuses on health inequalities as mediated by economic class. A wealth of literature also reports on health inequities as mediated by gender, ethnic group, and geography, but space is insufficient to do justice to the other variables reflecting social-group differences.

> **Box 2.1**
>
> ### Equality versus equity
>
> > If health is a critical component of human well-being, with which most will agree, one wonders why inequality of health should not be considered intrinsically important, independent of its correlation with other components of well-being.
> >
> > (Murray et al. 1999)
>
> In line with this argument, The World Health Organization (WHO) has taken the stance that one of the intrinsic goals of a health system is to ensure an equal distribution of health, in this case measured by disability-adjusted life expectancies (WHO 2000d). Figure 2.1, for example, graphs the distribution of life expectancies of males in Japan, Mexico, and the United States, with the United States showing a more unequal distribution. This, in and of itself, is cause for concern, according to WHO. The goal is to narrow the base of the distribution curve. Others argue that it is the systematic differences in health that matter and that these should be addressed explicitly in policy (Braveman 2000). The WHO analytical approach does not preclude the study of systematic differences resulting from social groupings (Murray et al. 1999). However, its specification of equal distribution of health as an intrinsic goal of the health system, rather than an equity goal, reveals an underlying philosophical framework different from that of advocates working directly to demonstrate and reduce social-group differences in health.

of quantity of life variously described in terms of mortality risks, life expectancies, and infant-mortality rates. Despite having equity as the overarching development goal, the Commission failed to define equity objectives precisely. Correspondingly, it failed to specify a way to monitor changes in the level of equity or what should count as a significant improvement in it if the Commission's recommendations on health research become policies.

EQUALITY OF WHAT?

What do we want equally distributed? Do we want to be equally healthy? What does this really mean? That we all have the same **quantity** of life? The same **quality** of life? Is this really desirable? Is this possible? At first blush, being equally healthy looks like everyone is getting his or her rightful claim from a just society. However, what would it take to achieve the goal of equal health for all? One extreme scenario would be that everyone values health equally and makes the same choices from among available health interventions. However, despite the availability of information on which to base their choices, people still have diverse aspirations and preferences. As Mooney (1994, p. 73) wrote, such a scenario is "too intrusive in terms of individual values."

Even if fully informed people freely made the same choices, not everyone would obtain the same outcomes from the same health interventions. The chances of avoiding death or decreasing the severity or duration of a disability through a given health intervention varies, depending on a variety of factors (comorbidity, severity of illness, and others). Not surprisingly, we come to the conclusion that health itself cannot be distributed equally. At most, the probability of obtaining a good health outcome through an intervention can be distributed equally.

Some people have translated this to mean that the goal is equality of access to health care and use of it. These are different but related parameters. When one is sick, one should have access to appropriate health care. *Access* implies availability of opportunity and is mainly perceived as a "supply-side" responsibility. The term *use of health-care services* goes beyond access and incorporates the concept of demand. But use is still measured in terms of the rates of use and is, therefore, still a resource measure, like access. Any straightforward link to health is missing (Pereira 1993). Some have gotten around this by attaching a qualifier: access to and use of health services "according to need." Fleshed out, this suggests the concepts of horizontal and vertical equity. Whereas horizontal equity requires the same care for the same health needs, vertical equity requires greater care for greater health needs. Again, on the surface, achieving horizontal and vertical equity seems like a laudable goal.

But what is need? Amartya Sen (1992) made the point that for true equality, it is not enough for society to provide opportunities (that is, for health care) for people to use. Society should also ensure that the individual has the capacity to convert an opportunity to its full potential benefit, if he or she so wishes. This has implications for a broader interpretation of horizontal and vertical equity. Given an individual has the same **medical** indication for a health intervention as another individual, horizontal equity demands that they both receive the same treatment. However, in Sen's view, if one of the individuals is not as educated as the other, for example, and is incapable of taking his or her pills as prescribed, then they should not receive the same treatment. This becomes an issue of vertical equity, as one individual has more needs, beyond the medical perspective, than the other and therefore should receive more inputs — not just health-care inputs. In a sense, this brings us full circle to the question of the meaning of equality of health, but this time, it is qualified to mean, equality of capabilities to achieve good health **outcomes** from broad health **actions**, not just health care.

EQUITY AMONG WHOM?

Resolving the issue of **equity among whom** means taking into account whether an inequality is systematically due to poverty, gender, racial discrimination, or other factors. Our choice of factors to explain differentials reflects our sense of **what is fair and unfair**, and this influences our interpretation of **how much inequality is inequitable.**

What is judged unfair will inevitably be contextual, but one helpful criterion, consistent with Sen's framework, is the concept of availability of choice. If someone knowingly makes the choice of an unhealthy lifestyle, then that is his or her free choice, and there is no unfairness if this individual obtains a lower health status than others as a result. However, when someone has no choice in his or her working or living conditions, then any resulting poorer health status or lack of informed access to potential remedies can be judged unfair in relation to any low health status resulting from a risk taken voluntarily and knowingly. More concretely, "the sense of injustice increases for groups where disadvantages cluster together and reinforce each other, making them very vulnerable to ill-health" (Whitehead 1992, p. 433).

The issue of how much inequality constitutes inequity is really the crux of the policy discussion. Ideally, this discussion should translate directly into a delineation of what ill-health is avoidable. This, however, is not an objective matter of deciding whether science is enough to prevent, remedy, or ameliorate ill-health. Rather it is a complex problem, oftentimes tinged with a sense of what is affordable or what is efficient inside or even outside the health sector (Ubel et al. 1996; Choudhry et al. 1997).

Societies will have to delineate clearly what ill-health they consider avoidable. For some, the health of the rich is an indication of what health is possible and, conversely, of what ill-health is avoidable. Others would prefer to set a minimum acceptable or adequate level of health and protect people's right to purchase services over and above a merely adequate level of health care (Buchanan 1995). Up to what amount should society pay to make effective medical technology available? How willing is society to address the other socioenvironmental determinants of health? This is the arena of competing priorities and difficult choices. A society's ability to **commit**

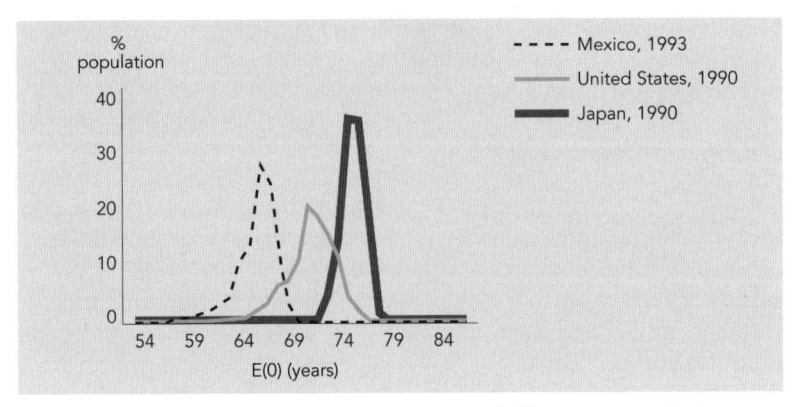

Figure 2.1. Population distribution by average male life expectancy at birth. Source: WHO (2000d). Note: E(0), life expectancy at birth.

to a realistic definition of fairness and of avoidable ill-health is what eventually distinguishes it from its neighbours who similarly wave the equity banner.

Equity in health thus implies a societal commitment to giving individuals equal capabilities of achieving good health outcomes, is conditional on respect for human diversity and individual autonomy, and is achieved through health action for the unfairly disadvantaged. Put more pragmatically, "none should be disadvantaged from achieving this potential [full health], if it can be avoided" (Whitehead 1992, p. 433).

CURRENT APPROACHES TO MEASURING INEQUITY IN HEALTH

When society has clarified its values and philosophical framework and committed itself to a definition of *equality of what* and *equity among whom*, it should translate the issue of **how much inequality is inequitable** into a set of equity objectives and initiate measurement, interpretation, and an action cycle.

Unfortunately, the choice of indicators for measuring inequity in health has often been limited to those commonly available: traditional health-status measures, possibly disaggregated by commonly studied independent variables. As such, the dependent variable of equal capabilities of achieving good health outcomes (equality of what) can only be approximated using health-status measures reflecting opportunities for health action and differences in human endowments and preferences. Such data include life expectancies, DALY, and infant- and child-mortality rates. Other proxy data include measures of access, use, or health expenditures. These are usually limited to descriptions of the financing, availability, or use of, primarily, medical care.

The dependent variables (equity among whom) have included economic status, gender, ethnic affiliation, and geography (rural or urban). They are available in the form of single categorical variables (for example, poor or not poor, male or female). Such studies therefore have two limitations. First, they give up valuable detail in the conversion of any variables with an intrinsically continuous distribution into categorical classes. As Sen (1992) observed, being classified as poor does not say anything much, because people have many levels of being poor. Thus, newer approaches have sought to describe health outcomes in terms of quintiles of income or wealth. Second, the synergistic effects of a combination of these variables in the same individual are difficult to tease out (for example, poor **and** female **and** rural).

Indicators of equity have sometimes been combined in a single summary index intended to reflect a society's overall equity-in-health situation. Bivariate contrasts (for example, richest : poorest ratios) are useful and evocative, as can be seen in Table 2.1, but they ignore 60% of the remaining distribution. Mackenbach and Kunst (1997) and

Table 2.1. Examples of measures of inequality presented by poorest and richest quintiles of the population.

Country	Period (years)	Poorest 20%	Richest 20%	Avg	Richest–poorest ratio
Mortality rate per 1 000 for children aged <5 years (Wagstaff 2000)					
Brazil	1996–97	113.3	18.7	63.5	6
Nepal	1996	126.8	64.6	91	2
Pakistan	1991	160.1	145.2	147.2	1.1
Viet Nam	1992–93	53.5	47.4	50.7	1.1
Percentage of those ill-buying or ill-receiving medicine when treated (Makinen et al. 2000)					
Burkina Faso (3 provinces)	1994	26	38	33	0.68
Kyrgyzstan (2 regions)	1996	8	14	12	0.57
Paraguay (6 departments)	1996	50	28	38	1.78
South Africa	1993	11	31	17	0.35
Thailand	1991	47	38	43	1.2
Per capita household spending on health, expressed as % of nonfood expenditure (Castro-Leal et al. 2000)					
Cote d'Ivoire	1988	13.4	6.3	—	2.1
Ghana	1992	12.7	7.5	—	1.7
Madagascar	1993–94	6.9	1.5	—	4.6

Gakidou et al. (2000) have been developing some sophisticated summary indices to fully capture the available information and monitor overall progress in achieving equity objectives.

As can be seen from the studies cited above, previous work on equity has used information collected for other purposes. Despite the limitations of these proxy data, compelling findings already show a picture of widely prevalent inequities in health. However, most studies measuring inequities in health are cross-sectional. No systematic surveillance has yet been undertaken of equity indicators that permit consistent time-trend analysis. A few countries are attempting this, such as South Africa, which has presented data by historically disadvantaged region (http://www.hst.org.za/hlink/equity0400.htm). The World Health Organization also started to collect such data in 2000 while monitoring the performance of health-care systems (specifically to study the performance in terms of the goal of distribution of health), and it has announced its plans to collect such data annually.

Recently, Gwatkin and Guillot (2000) reexamined the 1990 Global Burden of Disease data and compared rates and causes of disability between the global rich and the global poor. They identified the global rich as the 20% of the total world population residing in countries with the highest income per capita, and conversely for the global poor. They showed that communicable diseases explain 59% of deaths and 64% of DALY loss among the global poor, whereas for the global rich they account for only 7.7% of all deaths and 10.9% of DALY loss. The poor shoulder 47.3% of total deaths resulting from communicable disease and 49.8% of total DALY loss from this cause, whereas the rich bear only 4.2% of such deaths and 2.6% of such DALY loss. Gwatkin and Guillot also looked at the poor–rich gap on the basis of differences in the two groups' age- and sex-standardized rates of excess death and disability.

The World Bank applied the same methodology of comparing the wealthiest and poorest 20% of the population but using another data source, the large-sample Demographic and Health Surveys run in 48 developing countries. The data sets for each country are available at the World Bank website for poverty and health (http://www.worldbank.org/poverty/health/), with data disaggregated by age and sex and quintiles of wealth (calculated as an index). The difference in the top and bottom 20% is captured using a rich–poor index and ranges from 2- to 10-fold.

Inequity in health occurs even in developed countries, such as the United Kingdom and the United States, where the major causes of death and disability are noncommunicable illnesses and the poorest quintile may comprise mostly the nearly poor or working poor (Marmot et al. 1997). Convincing evidence of this phenomenon is also seen in the Whitehall study of British civil servants, which demonstrated health gradients with increasing employment grade within the British bureaucracy (as a socioeconomic measure) (Marmot and Shipley 1996).

LINKING POVERTY, INEQUITY, AND ILL-HEALTH

It is no surprise that poverty leads to ill-health through sheer material deprivation and that this initiates a vicious cycle. A study conducted in a village in Guinea (Evans 1989, cited in Sköld 1999) on the impact of onchocerciasis (river blindness) traced the disabling impact of this disease with time on individuals, households, and villages (see Box 2.2). A young man becomes vulnerable and exposed to

---

Box 2.2

Onchocerciasis: a downward spiral

— Onset of blindness due to onchocerciasis
— Increased dependency ratios (ratio of number of consuming household members to number of active producing household members)
— Decrease in nutritional and health status of all household members and increased vulnerability to other diseases
— Decreasing labour input
— Decreasing capacity to participate in traditional labour exchange system
— Decreasing area under cultivation
— Decreasing ability of household food production to feed household members
— Increasing duration of food shortage
— Decreasing ability to undertake food shortage coping strategies
— Increasing expenditures using scarce household resources on health problems, in particular blindness
— Decreasing household viability
— Increasing stress and household disunity
— Increasing reliance on village welfare system and extended family.

Although onchocerciasis may be on the verge of elimination now, the same cascade of events is easily recognizable in many diseases.

Source: Sköld (1999, p. 16).

onchocerciasis. Being poor, he has no access to treatment for the infection — and cannot afford it — and thus suffers the complications of the disease.

More recently, proponents of a relative-income hypothesis have presented empirical evidence to show that not only a person's income but also the distribution of income within a society affects the health of individuals. Thus, a socioeconomic gradient has an independent effect over and above the absolute impact of material deprivation (Wilkinson 1992). Using the Robin-Hood Index, which is the proportion of aggregate income to be redistributed from the rich to the poor for equality of income to be achieved, Kennedy et al. (1996) showed that a 1% rise in this index is associated with an excess mortality of 21.7 deaths per 100 000 population ($P < 0.05$).

Much of the analytical work uses data from developed countries. In a sense, the data show that the availability and use of health care in these countries can only partially ameliorate the effects of inequities, not prevent them. Even with universal access to health care, health differentials will persist unless we more fully elucidate and address the mechanisms through which socioeconomic gradients exert their impacts on health.

The loss of social capital, or social cohesion and solidarity, with increasingly steep socioeconomic gradients, has been postulated as a link between poverty, inequity, and ill-health (Kawachi and Kennedy 1997). Social capital has been formally defined as "those features of social organization, such as networks, norms, and trust, that facilitate co-ordination and co-operation for mutual benefit" (Putnam et al. 1993, cited in Harrison 1999, p. 132). The social consequences of income inequality are thought to be mediated through residential segregation, as exemplified in the "concentration" of disadvantages for those living in a ghetto (Kawachi and Kennedy 1997).

A recent work of the World Bank, *Voices of the Poor*, consistently echoed this message, expanding the meaning of poverty beyond lack of material goods and providing a graphic example of the loss of social solidarity (http://www.worldbank.org/poverty/voices/listen-findings.htm#6):

> No one helps, not anyone. I would gladly help someone, but how when I am in need of help myself. This is misery (jad). Our souls, our psyches are dead.
> — Vares, Bosnia and Herzegovina

Some data from ecological studies also demonstrate the relationship between social capital and health. For example, a study conducted by Kawachi et al. (1997) of 38 states in the United States correlates overall mortality ($r = 0.4$, $P < 0.01$) with the "withering" of social capital, as measured in civic distrust (revealed through a survey) and a low density of people's participation in community organizations.

MAKING EQUITY A PRIORITY IN HEALTH

Since the Commission published its report in 1990 no one has made any systematic effort to monitor changes in inequities in health on an international scale, much less to demonstrate causality and show how health research has had an impact on health inequities. However, some important regional initiatives are under way, such as the Southern African Regional Network on Equity in Health (EQUINET) (see Box 2.3).

A major stumbling block in many countries has been a reluctance to explicitly define *inequity* for their societies or, more practically, *unacceptable inequality*. Accordingly, none have set equity objectives or made a political commitment to addressing and monitoring inequities in health.

In the intervening years since the report, researchers have nonetheless made progress in demonstrating the prevalence of inequities in health, measured through either proxies (like health status, access to and use of health services) or expenditures. A number of studies have consistently revealed the inequities between rich and poor across countries, developing or developed, or within countries. Other studies have demonstrated inequities in health by gender, ethnic grouping, or geography. Equally important work has gone into elucidating the mechanism through which the socioeconomic gradient affects health. Even if a full causal model still has to be worked through and validated, researchers have made several proposals to expand the biomedical model of health to a social one. This model is fully compatible with Sen's notion of equality of capabilities. Old and familiar truths are resurrected in the social model, but it buttresses these with an expanded body of evidence.

Two of these truths are summarized below:

1. The welfare of the community is as important as the health of the individual —

    In many traditional African cultures, and certainly in Bantu culture, the individual does not take his or her autonomy from "cogito, ergo sum" (I think, therefore I am), as in the West, but from "Sumus, ergo sum (We are, therefore I am) — membership in an intensely important group that enhances the individual" (Nasseem 1992). Some Bantu words reflecting

Box 2.3

EQUINET: Exploring inequity in health in southern Africa

> Efficiency driven perspectives have dominated international health policy debates, and focused attention away from issues of relevance, of services as they interface with communities, or of how resources are allocated to these levels.
>
> — Dr Rene Loewenson, EQUINET Coordinator

Concern that the recent push for more efficient management in health services has done more harm than good — exacerbating inequity — is the driving force behind the formation of the Southern African Regional Network on Equity in Health (EQUINET).

EQUINET is a network of institutions and individuals working on equity in health in southern Africa. Its aims are to

— Further the conceptual framework and policy issues in relation to equity in health in southern Africa;

— Gather and analyze information to support scientific debate and decisions on equity in health in southern Africa;

— Engage stakeholders and, in particular, those social groups whose interests would be better served by more effective pursuit of equity measures in health; and

— Use all of the above to provide input into policies affecting health at the national level and the Southern African Development Community regional level.

Defining priorities of EQUINET include exploration of

— The extent to which various groups of people in the region can make choices about health inputs, the extent to which they have the capacity to use these choices for health, and the manner in which policies and measures affect such capacities; and

— The extent to which various groups of people have the opportunity to participate, the extent to which they have the power to direct resources toward their health needs, and the policies that influence this.

Financial support for the EQUINET project is provided by the International Development Research Centre. The Network is guided by a steering committee consisting of representatives from Botswana, South Africa, Tanzania, Zambia, and Zimbabwe and involves collaboration with colleagues in Sweden and the United Kingdom. Its Coordinator is Dr Rene Loewenson, Director of the Training and Research Support Centre in Zimbabwe. For more information, see http://www.equinet.org.

this spirit are "uglolana" or building each other and "uakana" or sharpening each other.
— Sen, B. (1999)

The social model of health recognizes that the upstream determinants of health (income inequalities, for example) are group characteristics and independent determinants of health. In this framework, health actions include intersectoral community-wide action to address the causes of inequities. At the same time, social capital can be built up by conscientiously providing opportunities for communities to participate in decision-making on what and how services (including health) are delivered and encouraging voluntarism in the actual provision of these services. "Average health is improved not by simply redistributing a given amount of health (by redistributing the current stock of health producing goods) but by reducing the psychosocial burden of relative deprivation" (Wilkinson 1997, p. 1727).

2. At the individual level, the interpersonal is as important as the technical aspect of health care —

In the hospitals they don't provide good care to the indigenous people like they ought to, because of their illiteracy they treat them badly ... they give us other medicines that are not for the health problem you have," says a young man from La Calera, Ecuador.
— http://www.worldbank.org/poverty/voices/listen-findings.htm#4

Within the health-care sector, efforts to address inequities should focus on improving not only the delivery and coverage of care but also its interpersonal quality. For example, care of a poor patient means not only addressing his or her physical problems but also ministering to the social consequences of poverty, vulnerability, loss of self-respect, and powerlessness (see Box 2.4). We also need fair financing of health care to shelter the poor from feelings of vulnerability and risk in case of severe illness.

This shift from a biomedical to a social model of health permits us to broaden the equity goal to include substantive and procedural equity. A society obtains substantive equity when it establishes an acceptable equalization of the individual's capability of benefiting from health actions, with priority given to disadvantaged people (whether these actions are intra- or intersectoral, at the individual or community level). A society can obtain procedural equity, or fairness in structure, process, or procedures to achieve substantive equity

> **Box 2.4**
>
> ## Health as a person's most valuable asset
>
> Invited by the Council on Health Research for Development (COHRED) to reflect on key messages for the health research and development community, Dr Robert Chambers of the Institute of Development Studies responded with the following observations:
>
> 1. For many poor people the body is their most valuable asset. It is indivisible and uninsured, which means the risks of damage or disability are horrendous for livelihood and well-being. With accident or illness it can flip from main asset to major liability for a poor household (it still has to be fed and cared for). Poor people are more exposed than others to risks of injury and sickness and are less able or willing than others to go for treatment and pay for it; and if they do get treated, their treatment may be less effective.
>
>   Message — Free, accessible, and effective treatment can be a highly cost-effective antipoverty measure. Enabling poor people to avoid becoming poorer is far easier than enabling them to struggle back upwards once they are poorer.
>
> 2. Many poor people do not go for treatment because they fear rudeness and humiliation from health staff.
>
>   Message — Training, encouraging, and enabling health staff to welcome poor people and treat them equally and with respect should be a priority within any antipoverty policy.
>
> 3. In terms of well-being, the opportunity costs for very poor people's time are often far higher than those of people who are less poor. This applies especially to women, who in the past decade have increasingly become the breadwinners for households. (This seems to be a worldwide trend.) Yet it is precisely those who are poor and look poor who tend to be marginalized in places of treatment and kept waiting while others who are better dressed or have influence jump the queue. For example, a poor woman who is nearly desperate and each day struggling to earn enough for food for herself and her children may starve as a result of being unable to earn while she is kept waiting for treatment for one of her children.
>
>   Message — Very poor people should have priority in treatment and at the very least be treated equally with others.

Box 2.5

Application of the social model of health: prevention of AIDS

Wolffers (2000) argued that there is a role for both the biomedical and the development paradigms in the prevention of AIDS. He warned against the biomedical paradigm dominating health action, such that AIDS prevention and control are viewed largely as a matter of developing a vaccine, providing anti-HIV drugs, and distributing condoms. "AIDS is at once a social and biological disorder; its course cannot be understood or altered without attention to its social and political context" (Fee 1993, cited in Wolffers 2000, p. 268). Condom use has been proven effective in reducing HIV infection among those who formerly engaged in unprotected sex. Those most vulnerable to HIV, however, are the ones in exploitative situations that make it difficult for them to use condoms. With this risk–vulnerability paradigm, "risk reduction programmes had to be designed and implemented in synergy with other programmes which in the short and long term, increased the capacity and autonomy of those people particularly vulnerable to HIV infection" (Tarantola 2000, p. 236). Thus, distribution of condoms should be coupled with improving self-esteem and control, strengthening social support networks, and advocacy for legislation to prevent harassment of commercial-sex workers by police and clients.

Preventing perinatal infection requires routine screening of pregnant women and administration of anti-HIV drugs before delivery. Women identified as HIV positive may be at risk of discrimination and outright harm if their HIV status is disclosed. Launching such a screening program means ensuring that, at the same time, an investment is made to develop an HIV–AIDS-tolerant society, where it is understood that "any member of the community can be infected, instead of isolating those who have been identified" (Wolffers 2000, p. 271). Support networks should also be set up in anticipation of the reality that even if the child survives, his or her mother and father will probably die soon, and society will have to care for the child, who may be HIV-free but left an orphan.

Wolffers criticized the consensus statement on preventing perinatal HIV infection

> that was published in the Lancet and was drafted by 11 authors, only 1 of whom was from a developing country, during a workshop with 40 participants in attendance and only 7 from developing countries. Including only a few scientists from developing countries in a consensus meeting cannot be taken seriously as a process of equal dialogue and should not be seen as a credible voice.
>
> — Wolffers (2000, p. 271)

Instead, he proposed that all stakeholders, including women (both HIV-infected and noninfected), orphans, members of the community who care for orphans, local health-care workers, and others at the grass-roots level, be included in a priority-setting and decision-making process to determine which interventions to implement and how to implement them.

(Aday et al. 1998), by encouraging participation in decision-making and empowerment through building social capital at the community level and improving the interpersonal quality of health care at the individual level (see Box 2.5).

It is fitting to end the chapter by coming full circle and quoting Dr John R. Evans, Chair of the Commission. He alluded in a recent interview to a possible way forward, in line with the social model of health:

> *The current analysis of how equity is achieved recognizes that the supply side is important (e.g. access to services), but one has to look also at how people view their own lives and how they can be mobilized to pursue equity rather than think of it as a passive concept.*
> — COHRED (2000d, p. 2)

POSTSCRIPT

The child with severe measles, whose hospitalization was paid for by her father's kidney, died.

CHAPTER 3

HEALTH RESEARCH: AN ESSENTIAL TOOL FOR ACHIEVING DEVELOPMENT THROUGH EQUITY

David Harrison

SUMMARY

The experience of the 1990s indicates that the Commission on Health Research for Development was correct in its analysis. Linked to equity, health research **can** be a powerful instrument for development. However, as long as market or scientific incentives are the only factors shaping health research, most breakthroughs will have little relevance to much of the world's population.

Drawing on country experience,[1] this chapter reviews recent thinking about health, development, and research. In particular, it places health research in the context of three major insights from the 1990s. First, the final nail has been hammered into the coffin of pure "trickle-down" theories of economic growth and development. Many agree that investing in health is critical to both economic productivity and human development. Second, events in this period have vindicated pro-poor, pro-equity activists. Countries with the widest gaps between rich and poor stumble along the "low road" to economic growth and development, handicapped by their own fractured societies. A common refrain from every quarter — from Michael Camdessus, director of the International Monetary Fund (IMF), to Nobel Laureate Amartya Sen — is that inequality is bad for the economy, bad for society, and bad for individuals. They each sing

---

[1] Country examples are based on case studies developed as part of the Health Research Profile Project (see Box 3.1, under "Getting the most out of investments in health research").

a different tune about what needs to be done about it, but the bottom line is that greater equity promotes economic growth and human development. Third, the application of knowledge is central to global development. People who used to talk about "established market economies" are now talking about "knowledge-based economies" — a change that goes beyond semantics. The use of knowledge is now regarded as the dominant factor of production in rich countries, surpassing even physical capital. The message promulgated in developing countries is that the route to prosperity is to adopt technologies from the North and adapt them for local use. In this context, research (as the basis for knowledge production) assumes even greater importance than envisaged by the Commission in 1990. It is more than just a strategic tool for effecting improvements in health; it is now the driving force behind all development.

Some have predicted that the new mode of knowledge production and diffusion will be the "great equalizer," narrowing the gaps between rich and poor. Evidence to date, however, suggests that knowledge processes, shaped by globalization, are widening income disparities. Although the motive for liberalizing trade and labour practices was ostensibly to benefit developing countries (through capital investment and knowledge spillovers), it has actually jeopardized the livelihoods of many low-skilled workers. Often the shift from labour-intensive to high-tech production processes has only made the problem worse.

Commercialization of knowledge (its conversion into a marketable commodity) has diverted human and financial resources away from the public interest — specifically, away from the concerns of the poor. Corporate intellectual property rights, embodied in multilateral agreements such as the Trade-Related Aspects of Intellectual Property Rights (TRIPs), may effectively shut out low-income countries from the knowledge-sharing characteristic of scientific discovery.

Whereas the Commission's analysis was accurate, its optimism was misplaced. The situation today is worse than it was 10 years ago. The Commission's report noted that only 5% of global expenditure on health research (which in 1986 was estimated at 30 billion United States dollars [USD]) was directed to research on the main health problems of 95% of the world's population (CHRD 1990). The World Health Organization's (WHO's) Ad Hoc Committee on Health Research Relating to Future Intervention Options conducted a review 5 years later and found that the situation had deteriorated — only about 4.4% of all public-sector funds for health research and development (R&D) was then going to the problems of low- to middle-income countries (Ad Hoc Committee 1996). Writing for the *Nation*, Ken Silverstein put it more bluntly:

> The drug industry's calculus in apportioning its resources is cold-blooded, but there's no disputing that one old, fat, bald, fungus-ridden rich man who can't get it up counts for more than half a billion people who are vulnerable to malaria but too poor to buy the remedies they need.
> — Silverstein (1999, p. 13)

Ten years down the line, then, we can say with greater confidence that investment in health is important, that equity matters, and that health research can be the foundation for better health. Yet, we cannot say that the world is better off for the strength of our convictions.

Can we improve the health of the poor in the face of a rampant international market and a preoccupation with research that only distributes dividends according to the ability to pay? A starting point in answering this question would be to understand why inefficiencies in public R&D allocations persisted through the 1990s, despite the recognition that health research can lead to substantially better health. One reason is that the international community failed to establish effective incentives to redress market failures, despite clear acknowledgment of the widespread negative effects of disease and the public good of health research. Multilateral organizations have responded inadequately to the prevalent incentives favouring R&D investment in the health of the rich, which, at the margin, produces progressively less health gain but more financial gain for both the scientist and the manufacturer. There are promising signs that this situation is about to change for the better: the new Multilateral Initiative on Malaria is an attempt to establish compelling incentives for greater public and private investment in R&D related to one of the world's worst diseases (UNDP–TDR 1999). This blend of public and private effort may precede a new type of international research infrastructure. As the distinction between science and technology increasingly blurs, traditional divisions between funding for public health research and that for private health research are breaking down. As a result, the international health-research community has an opportunity to better integrate the efforts of public, private, and nongovernmental organizations.

Yet, international incentives on their own will not bring about the required changes, and countries need to make a far more deliberate effort to put health research to better use. A number of countries have identified national health priorities and tried to set research agendas accordingly. However, even if investments in R&D do address national priorities, they may fail to realize expected benefits if the type of research conducted does not match the country's needs. For instance, it is not unusual for exploratory studies to dominate the research portfolios of low-income countries at times when the most pressing needs are to solve practical problems, reduce inefficiencies in existing interventions, and better allocate resources. The point is that the strategic emphasis of a country's research portfolio should reflect an appropriate balance between short- and long-term problem-solving and between the demands of helping to develop new tools, using existing ones better, and allocating resources more fairly. Low-income countries can realize greater returns on investment in R&D by better aligning expenditures with national priorities and investing in the most appropriate types of R&D.

A helpful metaphor is to think of the national research agenda as a diversified investment portfolio that aims to maximize expected social benefit. However, even if countries adopt an investment portfolio to generate the greatest improvement in health, they will only realize the benefits if they implement research efficiently, enhancing outputs and reducing costs. To date, much of the effort has focused on supply-side strategies to enhance outputs by building up resources for R&D. Less attention has gone to improving supply through better use of existing resources. Even more significant is the neglect of strategies to stimulate a demand for research, although they hold the key to substantial gains in efficiency. We are also seeing a growing awareness of the costs of some research being unnecessarily high, particularly in communicating information. Reducing these costs can substantially increase returns on investment in research.

For low-income countries, *returns* should be defined in terms of a better health status for those who need it most. Although R&D helps to stimulate a country's educational system and may in the long term contribute to economic productivity, these welfare effects are insufficient to justify investments in health research. Faced with considerable unmet basic needs, a country can only justify research if it leads to better health now.

THREE INSIGHTS FROM THE 1990s

INVESTING IN HEALTH IS CRITICAL FOR BOTH ECONOMIC GROWTH AND HUMAN DEVELOPMENT

By the end of the 1980s, the trickle-down–bottom-up debate had already lost steam, overtaken by mounting evidence (from failed structural-adjustment programs) that pure trickle-down strategies do not bring about the productivity gains expected, let alone reduce poverty. As a result, in the 1990s development thinkers adopted a more sophisticated theory, expressed in terms such as "structural adjustment with a human face," "high-quality economic growth," "smart growth," and "human development," terms coined by multilateral organizations. Regardless of ideological standpoint, the bottom line was clear. Without strategies to promote health, education, and economic security for the poorest people, efforts to foster productivity growth would be unlikely to bring about sustained national development.

The development community learned this hard lesson at the expense of the poor. Conventional wisdom held that productivity growth would significantly reduce extreme poverty. For instance, World Bank econometric studies projected that a 3% rate of growth per capita would typically bring about a 6–10% reduction in the proportion of the population living on less than 1 USD/day. Yet, a 1994 comparison of trends in 44 developing countries found that global poverty fell only slightly after 1980, despite positive growth rates overall (Ravallion 1995). The incidence of absolute poverty in the developing world remained static in the latter part of the 1980s, with one in three people living on less than 1 USD/day, and two in three living on less than 2 USD/day. In absolute numbers, poverty was generally rising in Latin America and sub-Saharan Africa, although the incidence was generally falling in Asia (Chen et al. 1994).

In South America and Africa, IMF economists were left scratching their heads about why policy advice had failed. In an article in the IMF journal, *Finance and Development*, Senior Policy Advisor Susan Schadler (1996, p. 14) wrote, "the most striking gains were on the external accounts; developments in the key domestic targets — inflation, investment and growth — were less impressive." If the key domestic targets of inflation, investment, and growth were less than impressive, the impact on the poor was disastrous. The economies of many countries contracted, reducing access to social services and further impoverishing the poorest people.

Worse still, the benefits of belt-tightening predicted for the "postrecessionary phase" of structural adjustment often failed to materialize. As Susan Schadler (1996, p. 16) observed, "for most countries outside Central Europe, there was some strengthening of growth and, on average, an increase in savings ratios. Still, no country shifted to a distinctly more rapid pace of growth backed by higher savings." Even where growth occurred, the poorest people were often worse off than before structural adjustment. In Argentina, Brazil, Chile,

Uruguay, and Venezuela, structural adjustment was associated with greater income concentration. Subsequent growth in the recovery phase did not necessarily restore income distributions to their former patterns. In fact, only Columbia, Costa Rica, and Uruguay (and possibly Mexico) returned to the lower, preadjustment levels of inequality (Altimir 1994). "Time," said the development pundits, "for a rethink."

For neoclassical theorists, this rethink meant elaborating on the importance of "human-capital formation" as a determinant of economic growth and human development. In the health sector, the landmark reference was the *World Development Report 1993*, which argued that a high burden of disease constrains economic growth by limiting human capital. Developing-country governments should, therefore, see efficient health-sector spending as an investment, rather than as a consumption item (World Bank 1993).

For human-development activists, in contrast, achieving good health was an end in itself and a good development outcome. The publication of the first United Nations Development Programme human development report, in 1990, gave credence to the efforts of development advocates over the previous 50 years. No longer was *development* synonymous with economic growth. In future, we would gauge national development on the basis of people's health and educational status, nutrition, poverty alleviation, security, human rights, and protection of vulnerable groups. Grass-roots activists felt vindicated: their efforts were contributing to human development — they were not merely providing relief and mopping up at the bottom of the pile of humanity (UNDP 1999).

At the other end of the decade, in 1998, the award of the Nobel Prize for Economics to Amartya Sen signalled a different form of support for an expanded definition of human development. His central argument is that development depends on the fulfillment of every person's individual capabilities (Sen 1999a). The persistence of inequality therefore acts as a brake on human development, and efforts to foster equality of human capability act as a stimulus.

Irrespective of ideology, commentators have agreed that investing in health is critical to both economic growth and human development — no stunning revelation to the people of low-income countries. In Côte d'Ivoire and Ghana, for example, 15% of the per capita gross domestic product (GDP) was lost to illness even before the impact of HIV and AIDS. Malaria and HIV–AIDS are probably the most obvious diseases undermining economic growth and human development. In countries like Tanzania, spatial patterns of poverty mirror the distribution of malaria, and the World Bank estimates that the direct and indirect costs of malaria in Africa stand at more than 2 billion USD/year. HIV–AIDS has substantially damaged economies in sub-Saharan Africa by increasing dependency ratios and diverting public expenditures from growth-enhancing investments. By 1989, the management of AIDS-related illness accounted for almost 70% of government health expenditure in Rwanda and more than 40% in Tanzania (Shaw and Elmendorf 1994). Economist Jeffrey Sachs pointed out that only three of the world's low-income countries lie outside tropical and subtropical zones, prompting his assertion that the best public-health intervention ever invented is the season of winter (Sachs 1999). This is not to say that Sachs implies defeat for low-income countries in the face of overwhelming odds. Breakthroughs against river blindness (onchocerciasis) in the 1990s have renewed optimism in the prospect of conquering other infectious diseases. We can achieve much more with better use of existing interventions — appropriate allocation of resources and greater operational efficiency (Ad Hoc Committee 1996).

At the beginning of the 21st century, the key message is that investments in health do not divert resources from the "productive sectors of the economy" but form part of the foundation for economic growth and human development.

EQUITY PROMOTES ECONOMIC GROWTH AND HUMAN DEVELOPMENT

How does health contribute to economic growth and human development? The *World Development Report 1993* (World Bank 1993) saw investment in the health sector as a way to reduce inefficiencies by bolstering aggregate levels of human capital. It saw improvements in health for poor people as a route to poverty reduction, by enhancing their ability to engage in economically productive activities.

An insight that has gained broader recognition in the 1990s is that it is not only the extent of poverty that matters, but its distribution as well. The implication is that strategies to reduce poverty should aim to narrow the gaps between rich and poor and not merely increase aggregate levels of productivity. Conventional economic theory has been turned on its head by evidence that high levels of income inequality constrain economic growth. Traditional views maintained that high inequality is an inevitable feature of some phases of national development (Kuznets 1955) or even that income inequality acts as an incentive for greater productivity (Garcia-Peñalosa 1995; Welch 1999). However, both econometric analyses and regional and country case studies have produced strong evidence that greater income equality promotes economic growth. For instance, greater equality has been a consistent explanatory factor in the economic success of East Asian countries, in contrast to the slower growth in Latin America and the Caribbean. East Asia had lower initial income inequality, and it had equity-oriented strategies of high investment in education and health, which paid handsome returns (Birdsall and Jaspersen 1997).

There is also growing evidence that at least part of the persistence of poverty in many countries is due to high levels of income inequality. Regression analyses have shown that initial income distribution is a good predictor of the rate of poverty reduction. A country with a low Gini index[2] (0.25) can expect a 33% drop in poverty rates as a result of a 10% mean per capita increase in gross national product (GNP), whereas similar economic growth in a country with high inequality (Gini 0.6) will reduce poverty by 18%. In fact, rates of poverty change are even more elastic to rates of change in the Gini index than mean per capita income: elasticity of poverty to the Gini index was found to be 3.86 (Bruno et al. 1998). In other words, seemingly modest changes in overall inequality can achieve a sizable change in the incidence of poverty.

Londoño and Széleky (1997), of the Inter-American Development Bank, argued that poverty in Latin America and the Caribbean is largely a problem of distribution, not of absolute insufficiency. In 1982, when the average Gini index for countries in the region was at its lowest, the incidence of poverty declined by nearly 2% for every 1% increase in per capita GNP. By the 1990s, the average Gini index was much higher, and elasticity of poverty to economic growth had declined: a 1% improvement in GDP reduced poverty by only 1.3%. The authors asserted that if Latin American and Caribbean countries had the income distribution of Eastern Europe or South Asia, they would virtually eliminate both extreme and moderate poverty.[3]

Simple mathematics explains the positive relationship between greater income equality and higher rates of poverty reduction. Given any positive rate of growth that is roughly uniform across all levels of income,[4] the poor will gain less (in absolute terms) than the rich. Higher inequality implies that the poor must have a lower share of the total income and its increment through growth, and at maximum

---

[2] The Gini index is a measure of income inequality, based on the cumulative share of total income owned by a cumulative proportion of the population.

[3] Extreme and moderate poverty are defined as per capita consumption of less than 1 and 2 USD/day, respectively.

[4] A reasonable assumption, as there is virtually no correlation between economic growth and inequality in analyses across countries (Ravallion 1997).

inequality (Gini index of 1.0) absolute poverty would be unresponsive to growth (Ravallion 1997).

Greater income equality promotes poverty reduction through other channels as well. These include a stronger political voice for those at the bottom of the income distribution and a weakening of the social stratification that traps poor people in the vicious cycle of low human capital and income (Bénabou 1996). "Polarization" is the growing concentration of very rich and very poor, and this appears to be the type of inequality that most constrains poverty reduction (Wolfson 1994; Ravallion and Chen 1997). This phenomenon has appeared at a global level in the concentration of the world's wealth in established market economies and the declining share of it in developing countries. Within many developing countries, the rich are getting (relatively) richer and the poor are getting (relatively) poorer.[5]

Another important insight of the 1990s is that it does not have to be this way. Some countries chose to systematically reduce inequality and poverty and prospered nevertheless. A review of 63 surveys from 1981 to 1992 (involving 44 countries) showed no systematic relationship between economic growth (independent variable) and income inequality (dependent variable). Countries were evenly divided between those in which growth came with rising inequality and those in which inequality fell with growth (Bruno et al. 1998). This finding suggests that government policies, rather than economic growth per se, determine distributive outcomes. Economic contractions have typically come with rising inequality, as seen in the recessive adjustments in Latin America and sub-Saharan Africa in the 1980s. But the right sort of government action can mitigate even this effect, as case studies from Latin America have shown. Altimir (1994) pointed out that countries consistently incorporating equity objectives into their policy designs restored lower levels of inequality, even in the recessive adjustment phase.

For advocates of human development, the maximization of the capabilities of every individual is a goal in its own right. They would argue that the painstaking (neoclassical) economic justification for a commitment to equity is unnecessary; nevertheless, it is once again relevant that many theorists and activists of diverse persuasions have converged on the same bottom line, namely, that equality is good for both economic growth and human development.

---

[5] This phenomenon is not necessarily detected by the Gini index but is demonstrated using the Wolfson coefficient of polarization (Wolfson 1994; Ravallion and Chen 1997).

APPLICATION OF KNOWLEDGE IS THE BASIS FOR ECONOMIC GROWTH AND HUMAN DEVELOPMENT[6]

A third insight from the 1990s arises from the evolution of "knowledge-based economies," with advances in information and communication technologies (ICTs) effectively breaking down national borders and radically altering power relationships between nation-states and global authorities. Some envision access to knowledge as the key to economic growth and human development.

Could the changes occurring with globalization in the 1990s have enabled low-income countries to "leapfrog into the 21st century"? Certainly the separation of finance from production suggests the possibility of massive injections of foreign capital into struggling economies; however, in practice international capital only flows among industrialized countries and a handful of lower-income ones (Bosworth and Collins 1999). Perhaps more importantly, many economists now regard the use of knowledge as a major factor in global productivity. Some have viewed the changed basis for economic growth as an unprecedented opportunity for developing countries: "regardless of current capabilities, individuals, firms, and countries will be able to create wealth in proportion to their ability to learn" (Johnson 1994, p. 23). Developing countries can now harness knowledge from anywhere in the world.

In the 1990s, economists and development theorists saw the use of knowledge not only as a way of promoting economic growth but also as a way of bringing about better social outcomes. For instance, the *World Development Report 1998/99* saw Costa Rica as a country achieving better than expected health, and to explain this it cited the country's policy of systematically disseminating and using health-promoting knowledge (World Bank 1999). In the words of innovation guru Peter Drucker, "the comparative advantage of less developed countries no longer lies in lower labour costs, but in the application of knowledge" (Drucker 1994, p. 53).

Yet, the role of knowledge in productivity growth and human development fits uncomfortably with neoclassical economic theory. For one thing, productivity growth occurs with human- and physical-capital accumulations, but independently of the invention of new technologies (Rebelo 1998). For another, the relationship between the application of knowledge and productivity growth seems to change over time (Nelson and Winter 1982). Innovation theorists have also

---

[6] See Figure A3.1, which presents a diagram and notes "mapping" the relationship between health research and development.

been quick to point out the shortcomings of thinking of knowledge as a tangible asset. Miller and Morris (1999) argued that knowledge exists only in people and has to be converted into new capabilities to bring about technological change, and Pfeffer and Sutton (2000) dismissed the notion that knowledge can be built up as capital stock, suggesting that it only has meaning when applied. McDonald (1998) maintained that, in the long run, the ownership of knowledge undermines the potential for discovery and innovation. Despite its uneasy fit, neoliberal theorists have conferred on knowledge a sense of fungibility — implicit in terms like "knowledge capital" and "knowledge spillovers" — consistent with the privatization of knowledge and the trade in knowledge as a commodity.

Furthermore, the "knowledge-capital" metaphor has reinforced the belief that free trade and foreign investment benefit developing countries. Some consider such activities good not only for productivity growth but also for knowledge transfer as a basis for economic and social development. Coe et al. (1997) found significant R&D spillovers from industrialized to low-income countries with low R&D capacities. Coe et al.'s regression analyses showed that on average a 1% increase in R&D capital in industrialized countries raised productive output in developing countries by 0.06%. Interestingly, though, the spillover effects occur mainly with arm's-length agreements, and there is little evidence that foreign direct investment promotes any efficiency gains through domestic innovation (Kholdy 1995; Navaretti and Carraro 1996). In other words, more knowledge-sharing and higher returns occur in low-income countries when foreign firms subcontract local experts than when the local experts are assimilated by the R&D machinery of subsidiaries.

Treating knowledge as a sellable commodity has also further accelerated the vertical integration of transnational companies trying to exercise proprietary control over every aspect of R&D and production. This is particularly true of the pharmaceutical and biotechnology industries within the health sector (Pisano 1991). Foreign firms have therefore had a stronger incentive to provide direct foreign investment than to establish arm's-length agreements in developing countries.

Low-income countries face a dilemma. Foreign investment has clear benefits in terms of economic growth and access to new technologies, but foreign investment usually follows the removal of domestic trade protections, which is not necessarily good for a country. Open trade facilitates the entry of transnational corporations into low-income countries, often at the expense of those with domestic innovative capacity. Liberalization has jeopardized the livelihood of many low-skilled workers and strengthened the hand of the intellectual and business elites in developing countries, particularly when liberalization means the removal of international trade barriers and the adoption of free-market approaches to labour supply. In consequence, it has often increased income and health inequalities, exacerbated by unequal access to ICTs (Lensink 1996; Ngwainmbi 1999).

Temple (1999) found it easy to envisage a hypothetical long-term equilibrium, in which developing and developed countries grow at the same rate after the developing ones have caught up by adopting technologies from abroad and investing in physical capital and education. But in fact, differences in rates of efficiency growth have widened between developed and developing countries over the past 30 years. We should look far more closely at our explanatory model before applying standard templates to low-income countries. Even if "knowledge capital" is only an analogy, we immediately run into trouble in trying to explain how the application of knowledge leads to economic growth and human development, because sometimes it fails to do this.

Impressed with high returns on investment in R&D in knowledge-based economies, some theorists have called for increases in developing countries' own levels of investment in R&D to enable them to fully assimilate new technologies. Much of the evidence for the theory linking R&D to productivity growth has come from countries at the forefront of the technological frontier, and there is little to suggest that developing countries can achieve the same economic returns. In the words of Nobel Laureate and economist Theodore Schultz, "even to be a free-rider requires a high level of scientific competence" (Schultz 1985).

In fact, R&D activities only seem to feature as factors of productivity once a country attains a threshold of economic prosperity. Using cross-country growth regressions, Birdsall and Rhee (1993) found R&D activity (expenditure) and economic growth positively correlated, but only across countries in the Organisation for Economic Co-operation and Development (OECD). (Even for OECD countries, there is no evidence that R&D activity **causes** growth.) In Birdsall and Rhee's study, R&D activities and per capita income showed a strong correlation, suggesting that R&D only gains in economic prominence once a country reaches a certain level of economic development. This is not to say that investment in R&D is unimportant in low-income countries as an impetus to advance science and education and address country-specific concerns. It does suggest, however, that the level of investment in R&D is an equilibrium state arising from both trade-offs and a complementarity with resources allocated to more basic needs. On its own, higher R&D expenditure in low-income countries is unlikely to accelerate economic growth or reduce poverty. We have little evidence to support the notion that the transfer of knowledge capital from countries in the North is somehow a shortcut to economic growth, substituting for other scarce factors of production. For low-income countries, a preoccupation with imported technology can, in fact, divert attention from the real challenge of putting local knowledge to work on improving social and economic outcomes.

This point is illustrated in the R&D portfolio Tanzania developed to meet its health priorities (see Figure 3.1). At a 1999 national priority-setting meeting, where research topics were scored in terms of priority, participants proposed that the bulk of national research effort be directed to achieving greater efficiency of resource use

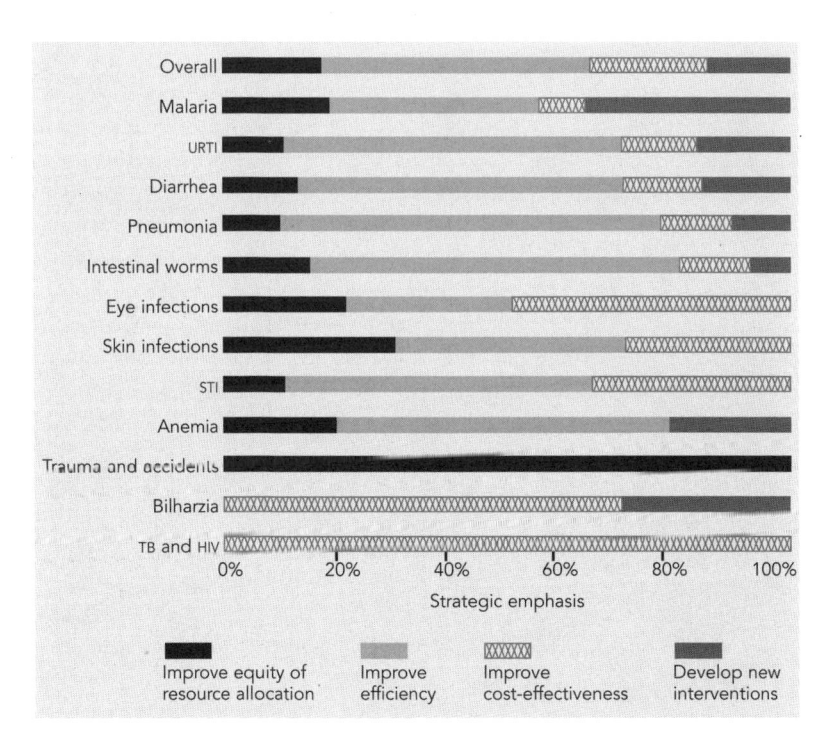

Figure 3.1. The Tanzanian health-research portfolio (placing greater emphasis on equity and efficiency). Note: HIV is not covered under STI. STI, sexually transmitted infection; URTI, upper respiratory tract infection.

(46.5%) or to improving equity of resource allocation (17.6%). They felt that less than a fifth (16.5%) of the national effort should focus on new-product development (Kitua 1999).

For the most part, developing countries require no new foreign technologies to improve equity of allocation and efficiency of use. WHO's Ad Hoc Committee (1996) made the same point. For many health priorities — such as acute watery diarrhea, tuberculosis, and pneumococcal infection — we would achieve the greatest gain at the margin by identifying and responding to inefficiencies in resource allocation and implementation (Ad Hoc Committee 1996). The main problem in addressing other health priorities is that the most efficacious interventions available are not cost-ineffective in low-income settings. However, local innovation **can** change the cost-effectiveness ratio, and developing countries can, themselves, certainly learn from each other's adaptations. Further, given existing technologies, a proportion of the current burden of disease is unavoidable, and to develop new interventions would require a global effort. The main reasons for persistently high levels of the most important diseases in low-income countries are failure to use existing tools efficiently and failure to allocate resources equitably. Sometimes, achieving greater efficiency simply requires political will and action. But often the technical inefficiencies and disparities in health status and distribution of resources need to be demonstrated. This knowledge can make the biggest difference in low-income countries.

Looking for foreign answers to these country-specific questions often leads developing countries to adopt inappropriate technologies and diverts even more of their resources away from their biggest problems. Foreign answers tend to be more capital and skills intensive and larger scale, require more foreign exchange and more advanced infrastructure, and often lead to cost-ineffective products (Streeten 1991). All this suggests that low-income countries can achieve the greatest gains using their own local knowledge and technology. Harnessing knowledge from foreign sources is an important but secondary objective, which is not to suggest that low-income countries would have no need to exchange ideas and technologies — it is a question of emphasis and the ways foreign technologies can boost local initiatives.

In this regard, the corporatization of intellectual property rights is an insidious threat to low-income countries, making it increasingly difficult for these countries to gain access to external information and contribute to global initiatives. The TRIPs agreement — administered by the World Trade Organization — requires signatories to apply the same principles to intellectual property protection as those governing trade between most-favoured nations. It establishes minimum standards of protection of intellectual property (including copyrights, trademarks, and patents), and it shifts bargaining power away from users of knowledge to those who generate it (often transnational corporations). As currently structured, it forces low-income countries to pay market prices for new information (UNDP 1999). This agreement has effectively pushed up the cost of acquiring information and has, indeed, been used to restrict low-income countries' access to cheaper health technologies, as when the United States was trying to restrict South Africa's access to cheaper medicines.

In many countries, rising costs have come with a decline in government expenditures on research. In Lithuania, for instance, the transition to a market economy has meant slashed public funding for health research. Almost all funds go to researchers' salaries and institutional overhead, and the research community in Lithuania is essentially in a "holding pattern" until the economy improves and more money is available for direct research expenses (Grabauskas 2000).

Much of the talk about the short-term benefits of global knowledge to low-income countries is more hype than substance, and the call for developing economies to "adopt, adapt and prosper" rings hollow for all the reasons given above. For most developing countries, the hope of fast-track development, or leap-frogging into the 21st century, is naive; slow but sure economic growth, accompanied by steady improvements in education and health, would be the most realistic basis for long-term development. Despite this modest projection, it is important not to lose sight of the real potential to improve health through knowledge-sharing and application. Research that really comes to grips with the specific health problems of developing countries and local communities can be a powerful instrument for development based on equity.

Investing in health is important, equity is important, and health research attuned to the specific needs of each country can improve health and promote development. The challenge for each country will be to ensure that its research aims for the maximal benefit of its people.

GETTING THE MOST OUT OF INVESTMENTS IN HEALTH RESEARCH

Even more so than rich economies, developing countries can ill-afford to waste their scarce resources. Yet, developing countries are the most hard pressed to demonstrate good returns on current R&D expenditures (see Box 3.1). We are also seeing a growing recognition that the conduct of science does not have neutral socioeconomic outcomes, and we need to scrutinize more carefully who benefits from "cutting-edge research" and whose interests are largely ignored in the dominant directions of science. The preeminent challenge for low-income countries will be to ensure that health research improves the health of the neediest people.

Conceptualizing the management of public resources for health research as a diversified investment portfolio is a useful way of thinking through the potential benefits and risks of every project. It encourages managers to work constantly toward better returns by comparing the expected benefits of diverse investment options (Eyzaguirre 1996), and it enables them to deal with the inevitable uncertainty of research outcomes by selecting a "risk profile" appropriate to their own countries. For example, an island economy like Mauritius or a small country such as Namibia (with a population of 1.4 million) would realize little benefit from R&D investments requiring large economies of scale. In this regard, Namibia's solid emphasis on problem-solving, particularly in trying to improve efficiency and equity in resource use, seems most appropriate (Katjiunanjo 2000[7]). In contrast, the wealth of Canada and the relative health of its population enable it to allocate more funds to exploratory research and less to trying to solve pressing problems. Yet, it can still have a portfolio designed to maximize expected social benefit (CIHR 2000).

Maximizing the value of health research means allocating resources to projects with the greatest expected benefit, as defined in the following formula:

Returns to each project under ideal conditions × probability of successfully implementing each study

Thus, even if resources go to the highest-ranked, "implementation-perfect" projects, one can expect benefits to materialize only with efficient implementation of research. In essence, then, maximizing the value of health research involves two iterative steps: (1) defining

---

[7] Katjiunanjo, P. 2000. Health research profile: Namibia (case study). Council on Health Research for Development, Geneva, Switzerland. (In draft.)

Box 3.1

Health Research Profile project

The title of the 1990 Commission report was *Health Research: Essential Link to Equity in Development* (CHRD 1990). The Health Research Profile project, sponsored by the Council on Health Research for Development, represents a step toward determining the extent to which health research has indeed influenced human development.

The objectives of this pilot project are

1. To determine the feasibility of using available data for the development of indicators for a national health-research profile.

2. To develop a prototype for a national health-research profile tool.

The longer-term goal is to develop a model to determine the strength of the relationship between national health-research investment and national human development. In so doing, it is intended that a tool be made available to countries to assist them in addressing key questions, such as

— Are health research efforts directed to the priority health problems of the country?

— Are countries using global and country-specific knowledge effectively?

The project was launched in 1999. Activities to date have included

1. *Identifying representative countries* — In each of four regions, three countries have been selected as representative of high, medium, and low human development, using the United Nations Development Programme human development index and its refinements. In addition to these 12 countries, three industrialized countries were also selected. The participating countries are Bangladesh, Canada, Chile, Ecuador, Hungary, Japan, Kazakhstan, Korea, Lithuania, Mauritius, Namibia, the Netherlands, Nicaragua, Thailand, and Uganda.

2. *Describing key profile elements* — Five categories of indicators have been identified, each with several subdescriptors:

— Amount spent on health research;

— Research done on health inequities (equity);

— Quality of research;

— Research capacity, and

— Research to policy, action, and practice.

3. *Determining the feasibility of obtaining data* — This phase of the project is currently under way.

The project team will be presenting preliminary findings during a special session at the October 2000 conference in Bangkok.

Further information can be obtained by contacting the project-coordinating centre in Ottawa, Canada: psquared@interlog.com.

an investment portfolio of research to produce the greatest benefit possible within budget constraints; and (2) implementing the research efficiently.

DESIGN OF AN R&D INVESTMENT PORTFOLIO TO MAXIMIZE SOCIAL BENEFIT

When designing an R&D investment portfolio, a developing country would have to determine three issues:

— Where to make investments;

— What type of investment "instruments" (for R&D) to use; and

— How much public money to put into each R&D instrument.

A number of countries have used priority-setting processes to determine where they should make investments, thus effectively defining the scope of research. For example, the Health Research Plan of Uganda (1997–2001) stipulates a clear list of topics as most important. These reflect the prominence of Uganda's health problems in the areas of

— Maternal and child health and nutrition;

— Water, sanitation, and the environment; and

— The communicable diseases of sexually transmitted infection, HIV–AIDS, and tuberculosis.

In addition, the plan circumscribes priorities for noncommunicable diseases and identifies priorities for improving health-service delivery (Okello and Emegu 2000).

The advantage of broad-based priority-setting over determining agendas exclusively on the basis of the prevailing incentives of science is that it better expresses aggregate levels of social demand (Dasgupta and David 1994). It also reflects the urgency of a society's need to address its health problems. In low-income countries, efforts to achieve immediate improvements in health care and other social services generally have high rates of return at the margin. To allocate resources efficiently, the public sector needs to use a high discount rate in estimating the present value of long-term projects. The implication is that projects with large short-term benefits are preferable to those with equally high long-term benefits. To some extent, broadly representative processes of priority-setting can reveal these preferences ("social discount rates").

Yet, even with valid priorities for disease research and appropriately allocated investments, research with a low expected social benefit may still receive the lion's share of funding. For instance, an esoteric piece of work on some biochemical change resulting from malaria may address a national priority, but it would surely fail a benefit–cost test. Even highly relevant research does not automatically pass muster. One should, for example, heavily discount the present value of future health benefits from long-term commitments to new-product development. In a country carrying a huge burden of preventable disease, failure to apply high discount rates to expected future benefits will result in an inefficient allocation of resources. However, the global investment in R&D directed to the diseases of the poor is pitifully low — about 4.5% of total public spending on health research (Ad Hoc Committee 1996). Even if every effort is made to use existing tools efficiently, without a stream of new interventions in the pipeline the future burden of disease may still be higher than expected. Malaria is a good example. Because drug sensitivities constantly change, new-product development remains a high priority.

So the next step will be to determine the profile of research expected to give the most benefit to each country. WHO's Ad Hoc Committee (1996) argued that disease persists for one or more of three reasons:

— Knowledge of disease processes and causes is inadequate;

— Existing "tools," or interventions, are inadequate; or

— Use of existing tools is inefficient.

The Ad Hoc Committee suggested R&D instruments to respond to these inadequacies:

— Develop new health products or interventions (discovery and invention);

— Adapt efficacious but unaffordable interventions to make them cost-effective (innovation); and

— Achieve greater efficiency in the use of existing interventions (implementation R&D).

In the Ad Hoc Committee's view, the concepts of both technical and allocative efficiency are implicit in the third instrument. It may be helpful, however, to more clearly distinguish between technical efficiency (putting inputs to best use, regardless of allocation) and allocative efficiency, defined by the Ad Hoc Committee as focusing resources on areas of greatest need. In conventional economic terms, we achieve allocative efficiency through market incentives based on people's willingness to pay. Using this term to refer to allocations targeting the greatest burden of disease may therefore lead to misunderstanding. But more importantly, strident and politically connected interest groups and a health-information system with a focus on wealthier areas are likely to distract attention from the very sector of the population most in need of resources. These factors make it very difficult to reveal the true distribution of societal demand, leading both national and global health-research agendas to substantially neglect the problems of the poor. Unless a research portfolio has an explicit redistributive component, the current trends will prevail. And so we need to add a fourth type of R&D instrument to the three outlined above, namely, achieving greater equity in resource allocation. For low-income countries, strategies to achieve greater efficiency and strategies to achieve greater equity in resource allocation will almost inevitably be one and the same. Without an explicit agenda for equity, however, inefficient resource allocation will continue.

It is important not to define "type of R&D" in traditional disciplinary terms, such as biomedical research, clinical research, epidemiology, or social science. To develop new drugs requires laboratory research, but new service interventions may also require health policy or systems research. Similarly, improving cost-effectiveness may, for example, require biotechnological innovations in existing diagnostic tools. Thinking in terms of disciplines rather than in terms of the purpose of research projects may lead to turf protection among researchers or a deviation from an R&D trajectory with the highest returns.

The final step is to decide how much to spend on each project to maximize social benefit. In other words, the research portfolio needs to become a diversified investment portfolio, one that responds to new opportunities as they emerge while taking account of budget constraints and existing funding commitments. Having estimated the direct costs of individual projects, one can then more or less circumscribe the range of feasible research options. Costing various research options may seem like a theoretical exercise to countries heavily dependent on donor funding, as their national research management bodies do not have control over most financing for direct expenses. Nevertheless, a portfolio provides a basic framework for financial management of R&D, which should help low-income countries assume greater fiduciary control over public funds. Without costing, the research agenda remains a "wish list." Without understanding financial flows, a country has no way of determining whether it is aligning its resources with national priorities.

The importance of this step is illustrated in the priorities chosen in Hungary and Uganda. Despite the value of their priorities, they were too broad for these countries to really direct their resources to greatest benefit. Uganda chose reproductive and sexual health in adolescents as a priority, and Hungary chose public-health research and epidemiology (Makara 2000;[8] Okello and Emegu 2000). These choices reflect the first step in clearly defining a scope of research, yet they were too ill-defined to ensure that resources would eventually go to projects with high expected returns.

A legitimate concern for researchers is that an overly prescriptive agenda may undermine the typical incentives for science, such as autonomy and curiosity. One option would be to specify a detailed research agenda but retain the possibility of funding for researcher-initiated projects. But these projects should still have to meet the criterion of high expected social benefit.

Before allocating funds to specific research projects, a country may set aside a portion of its total health-research budget for baseline institutional funding. Although competitive funding encourages diversity and discovery and is a mechanism for aligning research with national priorities, 100% competition is probably not a good option for most countries. A fragile R&D infrastructure will be intolerant to dramatic fluctuations in funding across institutions from year to year. National research capacity, already weak in certain disciplines, may be severely jeopardized if even one institution fails to secure adequate funding for a relatively short time. Although baseline funding for institutions may act as a drag on incentives to do good research, a degree of stability and security may also encourage researchers to take risks (Dasgupta and David 1994), and it may reduce destructive rivalry between organizations. A feasible alternative would be to have a mix of baseline funding for indirect costs of maintaining a research institution and a competitive system for direct investments in research. Research leadership requires considerable creativity and skill to manage the interface between competition and collaboration to ensure that scientists have incentives for both individual and collective innovation.

---

[8] Makara, P. 2000. Health research profile: Hungary (case study). Council on Health Research for Development, Geneva, Switzerland. (In draft.)

With further refinement, the investment portfolio may enable planners to anticipate future health problems, exploit transient opportunities with high expected benefits, or "sunset" less relevant projects. Revenue centres should be in place to channel funds for direct costs and allow monitoring of financial flows.

Each country would have to decide on its own strategic emphasis, and the resultant R&D profile would have to include ballpark estimates for the allocation of public funds across investment strategies. For example, warning bells should sound if there is overwhelming agreement that the country's priority is to improve the efficiency of existing interventions while most resources are going to developing new ones. Although practical considerations would shape the final investment portfolio, it should bear a close resemblance — both in scope and in strategic emphasis — to priorities expected to maximize social benefit. Even if the research agenda aims at the greatest social returns, poor implementation of the research program would eliminate much of its potential gain.

IMPLEMENTING A NATIONAL HEALTH R&D-INVESTMENT PORTFOLIO EFFICIENTLY

The efficient implementation of the R&D portfolio means

— Enhancing research outputs; and

— Reducing the costs of research.

For the purpose of this discussion, research outputs are enhanced if they lead to greater social benefit (holding costs constant). The gist of the following argument is that far greater effort should be made to stimulate the demand for research. Considerable potential also exists to bolster supply, simply by reallocating and leveraging existing resources.

Gibbons et al. (1994) remarked that research has, if not a standard, then nevertheless a "social" market, in which various types of consumers use the outputs of researchers. A supply-driven model lies behind much of the research in low-income countries. Using this model, these countries' policymakers assume that if they can train enough researchers and build enough institutional capacity, outputs will be put to good use. An implicit assumption of supply-side strategies is that market-driven (economic) incentives will provide the impetus for innovation once critical research mass has been achieved.

This approach draws on the conventional economic wisdom that the main market failure in R&D is underinvestment in basic research, because basic research has no obvious commercial application and therefore requires public financing (Pavitt 1991). Yet, in low-income countries, underinvestment in "upstream" research is not the only "market failure" — the demand for research expected to meet an enhanced supply often fails to materialize (Alvendia 1985; Bhagavan 1992). Public officials, the media, industry, community groups, and other potential users rarely seize opportunities to capitalize on new knowledge, and this weak demand is reflected in low national investments in R&D, low salaries for researchers, and limited use of research findings. Newly trained researchers find little incentive to remain in universities or other public research centres. Those who do remain find it difficult to sustain their enthusiasm for life-long learning and innovation, and many settle into a bureaucratic mode of work, with little potential for new discovery, and this further suppresses the aggregate demand for research (Acemoglu 1997). Supply-side capacity-building strategies that do nothing to stimulate the demand for research are unlikely to achieve expected results and may actually further distort allocations by creating incentives among scientists for private gain. Without public demand for useful research, efforts to strengthen institutions may only help to create personal empires, and funds to foster individual incentive may only lead to the self-aggrandizement of researchers.

Bowles and Gintis (1996) referred to this mismatch between supply and demand as "coordination failure." Innovation theorists echo this charge of disequilibrium, describing inefficient research as uncoordinated "pushing and pulling" — being tugged in different directions by the respective motivations of researchers and users. Researchers "push" R&D in the direction of their own interests and scientific incentives. Market-oriented users "pull" research in the direction of applications they expect to yield the highest returns. In this situation, research leadership can be instrumental in efficiently integrating push and pull (Baskerville and Pries-Heje 1997).

What does it mean, in practice, to stimulate demand for research? Science and technology (S&T) managers have traditionally focused on detailed financial, physical, and human-resource planning: How many researchers do we need? What institutional capacity is required? What level of investment in R&D is sufficient? Now we are realizing that the main purpose of research leadership is to stimulate interaction among researchers and between researchers and users (Segal 1987; Neufeld et al. 1995). For a small island like Mauritius, the need to engineer interaction between researchers and users is not a great issue: scarcity of human resources leads to the multitasking of individuals, who often wear the hats of researcher and service manager interchangeably (Mohabeer 2000[9]). But bigger countries need to make a deliberate effort to forge links between people traditionally working in separate spheres. Lithuania, for example, explicitly designed its National Health Program to integrate health care, research, and teaching. Synthesized research findings are a regular input into the design and monitoring of the National Health Program, and these findings are presented to plenary sessions of parliament (Grabauskas 2000).

In other countries, pressing problems have provided the impetus for demand-driven research. For example, Thailand's concern over high concentrations of iodine in salt led to a new low-cost technique to measure iodine levels, and government efforts to reduce the purchasing cost of medicine resulted in an effective new scheme for drug procurement (Sitti-Amorn 2000[10]). In Bangladesh, research is an important part of the Integrated Nutrition Program, accounting for 28% of the total public expenditure on health R&D. Its clear goal is to improve nutrition (Bhuiya 2000[11]).

In time, demand-induced research should translate into a greater benefit to society, as well as to researchers. As researchers' salaries increase, so will the cost to society of their research. But additional public benefits outweigh these costs — a win–win situation.

Nurturing the supply of health research is an important way to enhance research outputs, but the focus of supply-side strategies is often too narrow. For instance, they often emphasize building up resources for R&D at the expense of allocating them most efficiently; alliances with international partners, to the detriment of national consortia; and leveraging resources only by gaining access to donor funds, without giving adequate attention to creating a synergy of national efforts. A different, entrepreneurial mind-set opens up new possibilities for low-income countries. This new approach views health-research leaders, not as information bankers, but as "knowledge entrepreneurs" who aim to squeeze as much social benefit as possible out of every rupee or shilling. We can think of these research leaders as investment-portfolio managers, whose tasks are to

— Constantly redirect resources to options expected to give the highest returns;

---

[9] Mohabeer, R. 2000. Health research profile project: Mauritius (case study). Council on Health Research for Development, Geneva, Switzerland. (In draft.)

[10] Sitti-Amorn, C. 2000. Health research profile project: Thailand. Council on Health Research for Development, Geneva, Switzerland. (In draft.)

[11] Bhuiya, A. 2000. Health research profile project: Bangladesh (case study). Council on Health Research for Development, Geneva, Switzerland. (In draft.)

— Seize on new opportunities for unusually high expected benefits; and

— Achieve economies of scale and risk-sharing through innovative partnerships.

By executing these tasks, research managers can add substantially to the value of current investments in R&D.

A recent report on health research in Kazakhstan illustrates some of the challenges in developing an entrepreneurial approach to managing resources for R&D. This country has built up an extensive and well-organized scientific infrastructure in 14 research centres and 6 medical universities. Akanov, the author of the report (Akanov 2000[12]), noted that despite sufficient scientific potential, Kazakhstan's research capacity fails to address the main needs of the population, and investments in underresourced areas of R&D could dramatically improve the efficiency of allocation. These would include investments in strategy development, health promotion, and a clearer analysis of the specific determinants of ill-health in Kazakstan.

One effective strategy for reallocating resources would be to design appropriate incentives for researchers to work on neglected topics. Although some researchers in low-income countries can compete internationally, most have low opportunity costs and lower salaries than other professionals in their countries. Given the poverty of these economies, the countries have little prospect of increasing researchers' salaries, so they need to improve the "psychic rewards" of being a researcher. However, individual rewards and incentives are difficult to institute and, in any case, incompatible with a team-based approach. Where interaction and collaboration among researchers are the driving forces for innovation, personal financial incentives may well be counterproductive, and team incentives would be more efficient (Gibbons et al. 1994).

Amabik (1999) suggested that the strength of team incentives depends on the

— Amount of challenge they give;

— Degree of freedom researchers have in the R&D process;

— Design of the teams;

— Level of encouragement; and

---

[12] Akanov, A. 2000. Health research profile project: Kazakhstan. Council on Health Research for Development, Geneva, Switzerland. (In draft.)

— Nature of organizational support.

Carefully designed team incentives can enhance outputs by redirecting efforts to create the greatest social benefit and improve the quality of R&D. In sum, stimulating demand for research and reallocating resources to maximize expected social benefit should increase the returns on investment in R&D. Another way of increasing returns would be to hold outputs constant but reduce the cost of doing research.

However, in real terms, researchers in low-income countries face higher costs than their counterparts in wealthier countries. These differentials may result from the various types of higher costs encountered in low-income countries:

— Financial costs (almost all financial transactions are more expensive);

— Economic costs (transaction costs are greater, particularly in communication and collegial interaction); and

— Political costs (researchers may incur personal and professional costs in societies that repress free speech).

Dasgupta and David (1994) argued that the main transaction costs in research are those incurred in communicating information, which is a point borne out in many developing countries. Their communication infrastructure is poor, and their researchers find it difficult to tap into global R&D networks (which have little interest in low-income countries) (Gibbs 1995). Furthermore, the shift away from the conception of knowledge as a public good to that of a sellable commodity is pushing up the cost of information. In real terms, developing countries pay far more than wealthier ones for the same information. Some communication costs are internal, however, and stronger interaction among researchers and between researchers and users would reduce many of the costs resulting from inefficiencies.

In Uganda, the Ministry of Health has recognized the need for a dynamic facilitator to bring together researchers, policymakers, and the public to improve health and development. The Uganda National Health Research Organization has responsibility for forging networks and effectively breaking down the barriers that push up the costs of research and place the country at an unnecessary disadvantage (Okello and Emegu 2000).

The Rural Advancement Committee in Bangladesh has recognized the potential of information-sharing to improve returns on investment in research. Its Research and Evaluation Division places increasing emphasis on information-sharing at field, program, and policy levels (BRAC 2000). It has tried and had success with new avenues for disseminating information, including field-level workshops, prominent bulletin boards, and the popular press. Although such strategies require more money, they reduce the real costs of research and enhance outputs.

CONCLUSION

This review of insights from the 1990s supports what antipoverty activists and community organizers have been saying for decades. We need to invest in the health of all people and reduce inequities that constrain economic growth and human development. In addressing these objectives, health research holds even greater promise than it did a decade ago, as the application of knowledge increasingly underpins global development.

The experience of the 1990s, however, suggests that this potential is going to waste in a world dominated by the interests of the rich. Prevailing incentives for S&T reinforce these interests and do little to improve the health of the poor. The task, for both national governments and the international community, will be to create incentives for more R&D to improve equity in resource allocation and efficiency in use. And as traditional distinctions between science and technology are increasingly blurred, it becomes more critically important to design a different type of international research architecture — one that combines public, private, and nongovernmental efforts for the sake of a common global good. Given the striking opportunities to attain higher returns on current investments in health research, there is no reason why other incentives should jeopardize the existing capacity of any research discipline. On the contrary, better alignment of R&D with expected social benefit should, in time, lead to stronger demand for every type of research.

Public investment in health research should aim to maximize social benefit, defined as better health for those who need it most. Developing countries cannot justify health R&D on the basis of its contributions to educational and scientific capacity alone, despite the benefits of basic research for the educational system (Garrett and Gransquist 1998); at the margin, investments in primary and secondary education will produce higher returns (Psacharopoulos 1994). Nor can developing countries justify health research on the basis of its contribution to economic productivity, despite the effects of R&D

on social welfare (Temple 1999). R&D only becomes a major factor in economic growth once a country has reached a certain threshold level of productivity (Birdsall and Rhee 1993). Low-income countries can only justify health research if it efficiently and equitably improves the health of their people.

APPENDIX 3.1
MAPPING THE RELATIONSHIP BETWEEN HEALTH RESEARCH AND DEVELOPMENT

Figure A3.1 is an attempt to "map" the relationship between health research and development. If health research is to be an effective instrument for development, we need to understand the mechanisms mediating its effects. We can then strengthen linkages that lead to development based on equity and counter the tendency of health research to favour the rich. Trying to depict the linkages between health research and development is ambitious and, some would say, naive. Trying to suggest causal linkages is fraught with problems! But we need to start somewhere and, rather like doing a jigsaw puzzle, begin to fill in the pieces as best we can. I have tried to summarize current knowledge (as I understand it) and give one or two references for each piece of current knowledge that I find particularly useful.

The first problem is defining *development*. Current approaches to this task come under four headings:

— Economic growth;

— Reduction of inequality (defined later);

— Reduction of poverty; and

— Maximization of individual capability.

The second problem is dealing with the complexity and iteration of relationships, which I have tried to simplify without being overly simplistic.

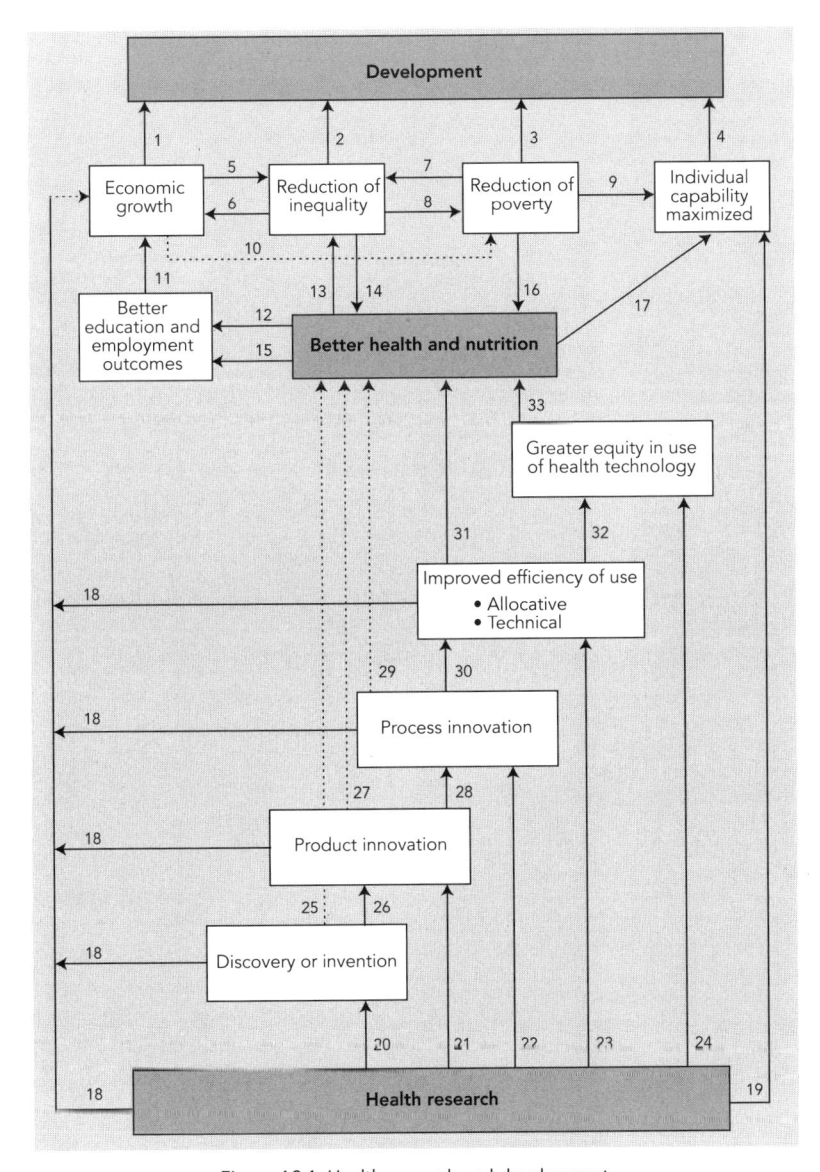

Figure A3.1. Health research and development.

Notes:
(1) Neoclassical approaches to development have stressed the fundamental importance of economic growth. This argument is well established and needs no elaboration.
(2) For those who view development as economic growth, inequality usually means *income* inequality. But it also refers to inequality in political participation, economic assets (land, human capital, and communal resources), and social conditions (housing, education, health). A distinction is often made between inequality of **opportunity** (lack of access to

essential inputs for productivity) and inequality of **outcome** (Tobin 1970). Others, such as Amartya Sen, see development as the maximization of individual capabilities. I have separated these two approaches, because they present different theories of how reducing inequality fosters development.

(3) Poverty may be defined in absolute terms (for example, the World Bank defines *extreme poverty* as income of less than 1 USD/day, adjusted for purchasing-power parity) or relative terms (for example, as a proportion of the median income). Relative poverty is a measure of income inequality, and the prevalence of absolute and relative poverty can move in opposite directions.

(4) Amartya Sen defined development as the maximization of individual capability through strategies to achieve equality and efficiency (defined in terms of "capability space") (Sen 1992).

(5) Econometric studies have found almost zero correlation between economic growth and subsequent levels of income inequality (contrary to the Kuznets hypothesis [Bruno et al. 1998]). In some countries, economic growth worsened inequality (many Latin American countries that undertook structural adjustment, for example). In others, income inequality decreased with economic growth. The implication is that national policies determine inequality outcomes, and governments can design strategies consistent with both economic growth and reduction of inequality.

(6) Econometric analyses, as well as regional and country case studies, strongly support the assertion that high levels of initial income inequality constrain economic growth. Possible channels for mediation include inefficient access to capital markets leading to underinvestment in human-capital development (Persson and Tabellini 1994) and sociopolitical instability limiting investment and saving (Alesina and Rodrik 1994). An additional channel is a disproportionately high burden of disease in a sector of the population leading to inadequate human-capital formation in this sector and decreasing aggregate productivity.

(7) Poverty reduction can also reduce inequality if targeted strategies reach the poorest groups, or if untargeted strategies benefit the poor more than they do the rich (Subbarao et al. 1997).

(8) Lower levels of income inequality occur with faster rates of poverty reduction (Ravallion 1997), and high levels of inequality can partly explain the persistence of global poverty (Londoño and Széleky 1997).

(9) The elimination of poverty is the central strategy for maximizing individual capability, by enabling individuals to reach their educational, health, and social potentials (Sen 1992).

(10) For established market economies, economic growth has been a major factor in poverty reduction. But the emerging economies of East Asia have helped refine our understanding of the relationship, and even organizations like the IMF now call for equity-directed economic policies (subject to "nondistortional" conditions) (Tanzi et al. 1999).

(11) Human-capital development, through education, and greater worker productivity are well-established factors for economic growth.

(12) The connection between better health and nutrition and economic growth is difficult to pin down (and is now the subject of a new WHO Commission). However, the *World Development Report 1993* and subsequent publications have argued that better health and nutrition improve educational and employment outcomes, leading to greater total-factor productivity (World Bank 1993; Temple 1999).

(13) Strategies that make the biggest inroads into global and national burdens of disease will almost inevitably reduce inequality, because they will focus on those people who bear a disproportionate burden of disease. However, global and national strategies aimed principally at marginal improvements in the health of wealthier sectors will worsen inequality.

(14) Conversely, strategies that reduce inequality (of opportunity or outcome) will almost invariably improve health status (through improved access to health care, higher income, less risk-taking behaviour, etc.).

(15) Better health and nutrition can lead to better educational outcomes for individuals and communities, which will improve their prospects of obtaining higher earnings. It should be noted that persistent social stratification can inhibit this outcome, by trapping poorer families in a steady state of low human capital and income (Bénabou 1996), even after health status has improved. Once again, this illustrates the need for equity-oriented development.

(16) The relationship between poverty reduction and better health is well established. Poverty is associated with higher rates of morbidity and mortality (Ad Hoc Committee 1996; Gwatkin et al. 1999).

(17) Good health and nutrition are prerequisites for the attainment of maximal individual capability (by definition).

(18) R&D drives technological progress, which in turn drives economic growth. Many studies have found high social and private rates of return on investments in R&D. Some have pointed out, however, that growth rates in OECD countries have not shown a persistent upward trend, despite accelerating R&D (Jones 1995). This is possibly explained by the growing importance of knowledge-capital development relative to physical-capital investments in established market economies. It is clear that R&D has substantial large-level effects on economic growth in established market economies, even though the relationship between levels of R&D investment and total-factor productivity is difficult to interpret (Temple 1999). There is no clear evidence that greater investment in R&D leads to higher economic growth in developing countries, and technology transfer from developed countries seems to be the principal determinant of economic growth (Birdsall and Rhee 1993). (Note that technology transfer is not a passive process but requires R&D [inventive] capacity [Helpman 1997]. The point is that targeted investments in R&D [as a way to achieve economic growth] are, of themselves, of little value in low-income countries.)

(19) New technologies and rapid knowledge development and diffusion create new possibilities for more equitable human development. They may create opportunities for individuals, communities, and countries to "leapfrog" many of the barriers to human progress traditionally associated with industrialization. But at the moment, the trend is in the opposite direction. Gaps between rich and poor are widening as a result of global patterns of investment. There is an urgent need to shape knowledge production and dissemination strategies to reduce inequalities (UNDP 1999).

(20) Discovery or invention of new health interventions arises from new knowledge of health and disease processes, and it establishes a dominant paradigm or course for further product development, process innovation, and implementation (Teece 1987). For example, the discovery of DNA in 1956 established a new paradigm for diagnosis and therapeutics.

(21) Once a dominant paradigm has taken root, product innovation tends to follow. The invention of monoclonal antibody (in 1975) and recombinant DNA techniques (in 1980) provided the impetus for further biotechnological innovation. New disease-specific diagnostic probes and therapies are appearing at a phenomenal rate.

(22) Process innovation concerns the refinement of the application of new tools (product innovation may be thought of as a refinement of the tool itself). Together, these processes improve the efficacy of interventions. An important implication is that learning (knowledge-sharing and assimilation) is a crucial component of R&D. Knowledge management strategies focusing almost exclusively on production will tend to have much lower expected benefits.

(23) The existence of efficacious interventions does not necessarily lead to effective outcomes. The report of the WHO Ad Hoc Committee (1996) showed that known interventions can avert a large proportion of the global burden of disease, but it persists because of technical and allocative inefficiency, or because known interventions are still too expensive. Country-specific political, social, cultural, economic, and other factors affect outcomes.

(24) Research that identifies inequities in health status and public-resource allocation and proposes and monitors strategies to reduce inequity can assist in improving the health of those who bear a disproportionate burden of disease (CHRD 1990).

(25) Some discoveries lead rapidly and quite directly to improvements in health, such as the discovery of penicillin.

(26) The persistence of communicable diseases like tuberculosis and malaria illustrates the importance of continuing product innovation in health research. New drugs are constantly needed to respond to changing patterns of resistance.

(27) A major concern at present is that the R&D "pipeline" of drugs, such as those for malaria, is almost empty (Silverstein 1999). Global repercussions are potentially considerable: reemergence of resistant strains of diseases in areas formally free of them and reversals in gains made in disease eradication.

(28) Biotechnology holds significant potential for process innovation. For example, diagnostic-probe techniques for a microbial infection like salmonella can provide a basic template for priority diseases in developing countries (Clark 1990).

(29) In developing countries, process innovation is especially important in achieving cost-effectiveness. Differences in the budget constraints of developed and developing countries mean that a group of interventions considered cost-effective in developed countries may be cost-ineffective in developing ones.

(30) Technologies are embedded in specific economic, organizational, and cultural situations. The real value of technology diffusion comes from using and combining technologies in various ways, not merely the passive transfer of information. Identifying the barriers to technology diffusion (often structural or organizational) in various settings is critical to improving efficiency (Watkins 1991). (IMB's "knowledge triad" is based on the integration of people, process, and technology [Cohen 1998].)

(31) Improved efficiency leads to better health by focusing public resources on people who bear the greatest burden of disease (improved efficiency of allocation) and investing in interventions with the greatest returns (improved technical efficiency). In developing countries, these are predominantly interventions to improve child and maternal health to reduce the current burden of disease, along with health-promotion strategies, like tobacco control, to reduce the future burden of disease.

(32) Equity- and efficiency-enhancing strategies for health in developing countries are consistent and usually reinforce each other. For example, allocating public resources for health care evenly across income quintiles (in other words, trying to achieve equity of access, let alone equity of outcome) would improve allocative efficiency. This would happen through a substantial reduction in the burden of disease on the poor, with marginal declines in the well-being of the rich. Health outcomes would be more equitable.

(33) Equity-oriented strategies enhance aggregate national well-being (reduced mortality and morbidity).

Part II

PUTTING COUNTRIES FIRST

CHAPTER 4

COMMUNITY PARTICIPATION IN ESSENTIAL NATIONAL HEALTH RESEARCH

Susan Reynolds Whyte

SUMMARY

Community participation in research and development makes good economic, scientific, and moral sense. It can, for example, achieve more efficient allocation of resources for research by better revealing the full extent of societal demand for various resources. Similarly, strengthened demand for research and interaction between researchers and users can make the conduct of research more efficient. Community participation also promotes equity by countering the tendency of research to reflect the views of an intellectual elite and by enabling national agendas to reflect the interests of local groups.

The community is one of three major stakeholders in Essential National Health Research (ENHR), along with researchers and policymakers. Yet, countries have run up against issues of who can and should speak for communities, biases about communities' ability and willingness to participate, and impatience with the time and groundwork needed to foster an effective partnership of all three stakeholders. Their experiences offer a number of lessons for realizing this ideal. These lessons fall under six categories, corresponding to the six questions addressed in this chapter, each of which underscores the need for considerable sensitivity, wisdom, persistence, and skill in appropriately involving various groups in research:

— *Who is the third stakeholder?* — *Community* can mean many things — for example, the inhabitants of a village or a group of geographically dispersed people suffering from the same illness or sharing an interest in a particular resource. It is imperative to articulate clearly what is meant by community while taking a pragmatic, context-sensitive approach to conceptualizing it. Community is defined for a purpose and in relation to other stakeholders in a particular situation.

- *What does community participation in ENHR entail?* — Participation may vary in intensity and with the phases of research. Effective community involvement is, most importantly, a matter of reciprocity and a continuing dialogue in which participation takes various forms and influences change in several directions.

- *Who speaks for whom?* — Elected or appointed officials, nongovernmental-organization (NGO) officials or front-line workers, health practitioners, and men often speak for communities. All representation is necessarily partial, but researchers should make it meaningful. Tokenism affects both the selection of representatives and the ways they participate. Researchers and policymakers have sometimes lost sight of the fact that ENHR inevitably challenges the priorities of traditional research communities; the politics of power ensure that the voices of the poorest people, who bear the greatest burden of disease, are little heard. The other ENHR partners must try to ensure that, in making their own voices heard, they do not make those of others less audible.

  Researchers and policymakers may strengthen existing forms of organization or help create new ones when they address some people and not others as representatives of communities. To address problems of inequity in health, one needs to determine who has not been getting their say and include these people in discussions. Without their participation, discussions of equity may remain abstract and academic. More importantly, one needs to create ways to view local realities from a national perspective — establishing a strong ENHR portfolio of community-oriented research projects provides the widest possible perspective. National research-coordinating mechanisms should establish guidelines or policy on the use of participatory methods in research and methods to encourage community participation in ENHR projects.

- *When is community participation in research relevant?* — Operational studies and action research have tended to lend themselves best to opportunities for community participation. They are as much about solving problems as about doing research in the academic sense. Joint explorations of local conditions by community members and researchers lead them to make systematic attempts to find new ways to manage problems. The research subjects appreciate this kind of "learning for a purpose." Yet, community participation is also relevant to epidemiologic and survey studies, as well as health-systems and clinical research.

— *What kinds of relations exist between researchers and communities?* — Community participation depends on relationships between researchers and communities, as well as on each stakeholder's expectations for the research. The issue of how researchers and communities relate to each other is also one of frameworks and institutions. One overall national coordinating body may not have sole responsibility for fostering such relationships. An ENHR mechanism should include the identification of frameworks to support contacts and strengthen the capacity of communities as users of research.

— *What are the expectations and trade-offs of community participation?* — Not always is there a synergy of interests among stakeholders. Community participation demands resources from the researchers, especially time, for dialogue and attend to the interests and expectations of community members, which often conflict with research goals or methods. Communities tend to be most interested in knowledge that has relevance to their lives. Demands are made on their time and material resources, often with no compensation. When their efforts seem to result in no benefit, they may feel bitter or lose interest in the research.

In future, it may be most fruitful to think of the relations among community, researcher, and policymaker as a coalition struck to define problems and learn ways to solve them. The rigid "iron-triangle" concept of the stakeholders, with its linear communications and trade-offs, should give way to an idea of learning and innovation coalitions that entail issue-based alliances, debate, and negotiation between sometimes disparate parties. Such coalitions draw on the knowledge and experience of all partners to define common goals, acquire new understanding, and develop solutions to specific health problems. They require flexibility and a long-term approach.

Instead of thinking in terms of conventional individual research protocols with set objectives, researchers should think in terms of phases of research, series of projects, or continuing exchange. To establish dialogue, researchers must meet communities in a variety of situations over time, so that they each have real opportunities to learn and communicate. It also requires researchers to communicate about their research in appropriate ways. Disseminating findings and improving the researchers' skills in this area are crucial tasks. Social accountability needs to be instilled in new researchers and encouraged in more experienced ones.

The organizations of civil society may have special roles to play in coalition-building. Structures need to be in place to encourage relationships between organizations and researchers, and here policymakers should take steps to establish an organ or channel of communication. A possible avenue for this would be what are known in Europe and North America as "science shops," which function as a link between universities and communities in the larger society.

Fostering an awareness of these obligations — along with the willingness of communities to take ownership of their health and well-being and work toward individual and social change — is the task of purpose-specific coalitions and the means to achieving greater equity in health and links between policy and action.

INTRODUCTION

Community participation in development activities has been a major policy theme since the 1970s. The emphasis on participation represents a paradigm shift in development work, an effort to reconceptualize the way planners address people and problems. Using participatory approaches, researchers have tried to put people first (Cernea 1991), or put the "last first" (Chambers 1983), through consultation, dialogue, and collaboration. The importance of this approach in the area of health has been clearly recognized, and the 1978 Alma Alta Declaration included people's participation as a fundamental ideal. Twenty years on, it is still considered an essential part of health development, but there is growing recognition that community participation is not a simple matter (Oakley 1989; Morgan 1993; Jewkes and Murcott 1996; Guijt and Shah 1998; Zakus and Lysack 1998).

The emphasis on participation in development work calls for a new approach to research. A whole family of techniques, known as "participatory-research" methods, has come into use. They have in common "a reorientation in the relationship between the outsider and the subjects of development activities and research: i.e. a reciprocal learning process in the relationship has replaced the one-way 'transfer of know-how' idea" (Mikkelsen 1995, p. 69). This reorientation is not merely about new techniques for gathering data; it concerns reciprocity within political cultures of information-sharing and dialogue (Pottier 1997).

A growing literature documents the experience of participatory health research (Nichter 1984; Seeley et al. 1992; De Koning and Martin 1996; Hardon 1998). Some of these studies refine tools for participatory research; some raise problems about what *community* and *participation* mean. This literature contains rich examples of the challenges posed by gender differences and power disparities. But what this chapter emphasizes are the more general issues about the politics of research: participatory research in health should involve dialogue about objectives for change and the research agenda, as well as involving an exchange of knowledge (Tan and Hardon 1998). These broader issues of reciprocity, agenda-setting, and mutual learning are highly relevant to ENHR.

In ENHR, community participation has been an important ideal in promoting health and development based on equity and social justice. The community is one of the three major stakeholders in ENHR, together with researchers and policymakers, and community participation is an important part of the ENHR strategy for action (TFHRD 1991).

How does community participation actually operate in the ENHR strategy? Is it merely lip service paid to a nice idea? How might it function? This chapter examines how people have defined, understood, and practiced community participation in countries trying to implement ENHR.[1] In particular, it uses the experiences of Bangladesh, Guinea, the Philippines, Trinidad and Tobago, and Uganda to highlight some of the key challenges in realizing this often difficult ideal. This chapter raises questions, addresses these questions, and proposes a reenergized concept of community participation for ENHR and for health research for development more broadly.

---

[1] The chapter is based largely on the report of the Council on Health Research for Developmemt's Working Group on Community Participation, which undertook a review of community participation in the ENHR experience of five countries (COHRED 2000b).

THE THIRD STAKEHOLDER AND THE ENHR STRATEGY FOR ACTION

A basic principle of ENHR is to create a partnership of three categories of actors: policy- or decision-makers, researchers, and communities (TFHRD 1991). Yet, who and what constitutes that third party? What does participation or involvement entail? Who speaks for whom? At what levels (national, district, or neighbourhood) can communities participate? When is community participation relevant and when is it not? In setting out the goals and principles of the ENHR strategy for action, the report of the Task Force on Health Research for Development equated the community with the public, the population, people, and users of health services. The report considered community involvement important in several of the strategy's seven elements, specifically promotion and advocacy, the ENHR mechanism, and priority-setting. However, it overlooked the potential opportunities for community participation in capacity-building and capacity-strengthening, networking, financing, and evaluation.

The Task Force saw community leaders and NGO representatives as possible prime movers, who would be able to promote dialogue at various levels of the health system and mobilize support for the ENHR concept. It recognized that political support for and the sustainability of ENHR depend in part on popular understanding and commitment. It also made community representation within the resulting ENHR mechanism a goal. The membership of the ENHR mechanisms should include representatives of public interests and concerns, such as individuals from relevant government and nongovernmental institutions, national health or population forums, women's organizations, and other concerned groups from civil society. Moreover, "changes in the management of research," the Task Force argued, "should go beyond cosmetic changes in the names and titles of people and programs — and beyond the token appointments of a few non-medical people to critical decision-making bodies" (TFHRD 1991, p. 45). It saw priority-setting, among the tasks of the ENHR mechanism, as the primary avenue for community involvement.

The ENHR strategy implies a new, open, and inclusive approach to setting health-research priorities. Such a strategy would take the community's perception of the importance of various problems into account, alongside epidemiological data on their magnitude, clinical measures of impacts on mortality and morbidity, and analyses of the economic and social costs to communities, families, and individuals. Given ENHR's focus on equity, one should weight the criteria for selecting priorities in favour of the poor, underserved, and disadvantaged sections of the population. In putting these principles into practice, however, countries have run up against the problems of who can and should speak for communities, biases about communities' ability and willingness to participate, and impatience with the time and groundwork needed to foster an effective partnership of all three stakeholders. The priority-setting process within various countries has been, in a way, a laboratory for community participation in ENHR. As well, research projects carried out as part of the ENHR plan have offered lessons on the nature and value of community involvement.

QUESTIONS AND LESSONS

An interim assessment of ENHR, conducted in 1996, found that "in no country [were] all three key 'stakeholders' (researchers, community representatives, and decision-makers) involved at every stage of the ENHR process" (COHRED 1996, p. ii). A review of country experiences in priority-setting revealed that the community is often dropped from the process in its later stages (COHRED 1997b). Considerable variation appears across countries in the extent of community involvement. Two country case studies of third-stakeholder involvement in ENHR appear in Boxes 4.1 and 4.2. They illustrate some of the many approaches various countries have taken in eliciting community participation. They also point to the interim-assessment team's finding that "the process of appropriately involving the various groups requires considerable sensitivity, wisdom, persistence, and skill" (COHRED 1996, p. 31). This chapter addresses six questions posed by the many country experiences.

WHO IS THE THIRD STAKEHOLDER?

Community is often used to refer to the public, or people in general. A community may also be thought of as a geopolitical unit. The term *community* can refer to the inhabitants of a locality administered as a unit, such as a village. Community involves common conditions, activities, and problems and often some sense of solidarity. One can describe it in terms of social structure (for example, local councils, schools, or numbers of households). As the Uganda case study reveals, a community in the geographical sense can be taken to represent community in its broadest sense, or the public in general. Hence, the popularity of the phrase "participation of communities," which covers both bases. Researchers may undertake consultations in a sampling of villages they think are representative of the community at large.

Box 4.1

Third-stakeholder involvement in ENHR: the Bangladesh experience

In Bangladesh, Essential National Health Research is firmly rooted within civil society. It operates under the umbrella of the Bangladesh Rural Advancement Committee (BRAC), the largest NGO in the country. Its activities are planned and guided by a working group consisting of 12 members, predominantly from NGOs involved in grass-roots-level program planning and implementation. The coordinator of ENHR in Bangladesh is also an NGO representative.

From initial efforts at promotion and advocacy to priority-setting and networking, civil society has been an active partner in ENHR in Bangladesh. Over time, people at large have been informed and sensitized through the mass media about the philosophy of ENHR and the ENHR movement in Bangladesh. A national-level workshop on ENHR — organized by BRAC, in collaboration with the Council on Health Research for Development, in June 1989 — was attended by 43 participants, 24 of whom were from various segments of civil society, such as women's forums, NGOs, universities, and autonomous bodies. A follow-up workshop, held 7 months later, supported a strong role for NGOs in government planning in health. When ENHR was formally launched in Bangladesh in November 1990, through a high-level national workshop, a press conference was arranged to explain the concept of ENHR to journalists. Many of the daily English and Bengali papers subsequently brought ENHR to the notice of the general public. Two issues of a newsletter on ENHR in Bangladesh, entitled "LIAISON: A Link Between Producers and Users of Health Research," were published in 1994 and 1996 and widely distributed to NGOs, special-interest groups, and academicians.

The 1989 ENHR workshop emphasized the need for a community-driven research agenda. Community participation in setting the national health-research agenda has been realized chiefly through civil-society representation within the Working Group, which is responsible for determining priority research areas. The community's perceptions of health and health problems, identified through various community-based surveys or studies, have also informed the priority-setting process. Under a capacity-building scheme, ENHR in Bangladesh contracted out 18 research studies to young researchers. The researchers gathered information from rural–urban communities. Some used participatory methods for gathering information. Though the interactions with the communities were, for the most part, of fleeting character, they provided rich information for understanding health needs.

Networking activities have included the formation of a broad-based, multidisciplinary network of 22 individuals from 20 institutions. Civil society has again been well represented. The majority of the members (59%) of this national forum are leaders of NGOs, health-related national forums, and women's organizations and senior academicians.

Source: Choudhury (1999).

Box 4.2

Third-stakeholder involvement in ENHR: the Uganda experience

From its outset, ENHR in Uganda has enjoyed the support of the Uganda National Council for Science and Technology and the Ministry of Health. Both were instrumental in its implementation, organizing a national ENHR workshop in February 1991. Participants at the workshop were primarily senior officials and scientists. Although recognition was given to the need to sensitize the community and mobilize support within it for ENHR, subsequent promotion and advocacy has been directed at research institutions, district health officials, and policymakers within the Ministry of Health and other relevant ministries.

When a national task force was created to consult on research priorities, a person from the Uganda Community Based Health Care Association was included to represent the third stakeholder. To date, however, community participation has been confined largely to the initial priority-setting exercise, undertaken by an ad hoc committee. This ad hoc committee engaged in separate consultations with each of the three stakeholder groups. Interviews were conducted with senior government officials and researchers. As well, the ad hoc committee visited three districts (Iganga, Mukono, and Hoima) and held a 2-day seminar with the district planning committee and the district health team. Some members of the planning committee were local politicians representing counties in the district. Following the seminar, focus-group discussions were held in one or two villages in the district. Participants in the village discussions included men and women, young and old.

Members of the ad hoc committee were impressed by the people's deep interest in discussing their health problems. Unlike the researchers, whose priorities were based on disease burden, the communities had a more holistic view of health and illness. All communities expressed the view that emphasis should be on not only disease but also fighting the factors that predispose people to ill-health.

Enhancing third-stakeholder participation remains one of the challenges facing ENHR in Uganda (COHRED 1997a). Given Uganda's policy of decentralization, the ENHR coordinating team is now trying to develop the capacity to set research priorities and carry out relevant research at the district level. This is expected to present greater opportunities for community participation. District health teams are encouraged to involve stakeholders in defining district-specific research problems. In several pilot districts, members of the health team are being supported to carry out such research, analyze results, disseminate them, and use them for planning.

Source: Neema (1999).

Examples of ENHR research suggest several other understandings of *community*. People who share a common interest, occupation, or cause may also be a community. Community in this sense has no specific location. Members of trade unions, linguistic or ethnic groups, religious groups, advocates of family planning, or patients suffering from the same disease, although they do not live in the same place, may nevertheless have a feeling of common identity in some respects. But they may or may not organize themselves as a group. Similarly, *community* may refer to people who mobilize around a given activity or resource. This is a more dynamic view, which recognizes that diverse communities come into being in various situations. What the individuals have in common may be conflicting interests in a resource, rather than a harmonious similarity of views.

In addition, researchers or policymakers may understand community to be the target group of a project or policy. When speaking about communities, frequently researchers, policymakers, or administrators refer to intended program or policy beneficiaries as "the masses," "the grass roots," "the poorest of the poor," the marginalized, or the users of health services. *Community* may also be shorthand for the subjects of a research project (for example, pregnant teenagers, TB patients). In essence, the community is that category of people that researchers or policymakers want to do something for, to, about, or with.

Community is a broad, friendly term, and loose concepts can be useful. But they can also become superficial and contribute to fuzzy thinking. For future ENHR work, it is imperative to clearly articulate what is meant by a community while taking a pragmatic and context-sensitive approach to conceptualizing it. Within such an approach, community is what community does. Community should be defined for a purpose and in relation to other stakeholders in a particular situation.

WHAT DOES COMMUNITY PARTICIPATION IN ENHR ENTAIL?

Community involvement can take various forms, including co-option and compliance, consultation, cooperation, colearning, and collective action (Cornwall 1996, p. 96) (see Box 4.3). In Uganda, for example, community consultation informed the national priority-setting process, and projects at the district and village levels involved cooperation and colearning. The question one needs to address in ENHR is what kinds of involvement are useful, efficient, or valuable and in what kinds of situations. It may well be that communities are more interested in the opportunity to learn from, and use, research than in

> **Box 4.3**
>
> ### Forms of community participation
>
> **Co-option and compliance**
> People participate by being dutiful subjects of research. They answer questions, keep appointments, give samples, and provide support for researchers in the field in the form of help with logistics, food, and shelter.
>
> **Consultation**
> The community is invited to present "the people's perspective" on problems of interest to researchers. This is usually done in the early stages of research planning and may be a one-time exercise.
>
> **Cooperation**
> Members of the community are involved in planning or execution of research, or both. They may have an influence on what research is done and how. In some cases, they help collect data.
>
> **Colearning**
> The community acquires new knowledge and skills from the research, either through dialogue or through being involved in the process.
>
> **Collective action**
> Together, the researchers and community (and policymakers) take action to make changes. Such action is related to research in two ways: it builds on new knowledge created by research, and the process of implementation itself is a learning experience.
>
> Source: Adapted from Cornwall (1996).

carrying it out. Yet, researchers rarely give feedback on their results to the subjects themselves or to a broader public. It is all too common to hear remarks like "a professor came here and took my urine — but we never heard anything more about it."

According to a linear and mechanical model of community participation, communities articulate their problems and help to carry out policy-relevant research. This "classic" approach has many variations (see Box 4.4), with participation occurring in various degrees of intensity and in diverse phases of the research. Most importantly, however, effective involvement is a matter of reciprocity and continuing dialogue, one in which participation takes various forms and influences change in several directions. People need information about research and policy if they are to be stakeholders in ENHR. Researchers have to work with the media, advocacy groups, health workers, and relevant organizations to make it meaningful for the community to participate in the sense of colearning and collective action.

> Box 4.4
>
> ### A middle way: participatory approach to improving newborn care in Nepal
>
> The classic grass-roots participatory approach is open ended, encouraging the community to define the problem to be solved. This bottom-up approach contrasts with the usual top-down style of health research, where researchers identify a health problem, suggest a solution, introduce an intervention to the community, and evaluate the effectiveness of the intervention.
>
> A project, based at the Institute of Child Health in London and Mother and Infant Research Activities in Kathmandu and financed by the Department for International Development, set out to test an approach that is a sort of middle way between the two with rural communities in Nepal. At the outset, the researchers defined the project's focus on neonatal health, but communities were encouraged to come up with solutions, with the help of trained local facilitators.
>
> The problem addressed by the project is neonatal mortality — deaths within the first 4 weeks of life. In developing countries, 7 in every 10 infant deaths occur within this period. It is a particular problem in the poorest communities where most deliveries occur at home. In Nepal, 95% of women deliver at home, where consequently the majority of neonatal deaths occur. Yet, many of these deaths could be avoided with changes in how newborn infants are cared for.
>
> Facilitators introduced the research to the communities and encouraged discussion about why newborn infants become ill or die. A shared sense of what should be done was developed, and each group set its own agenda of activities. Changes in practice were intended to be self-sustaining, and women were identified within the community to act as leaders and maintain the impetus for change after the researchers left the field.
>
> Source: Costello (2000).

WHO SPEAKS FOR WHOM?

The level of community involvement in planning and action may be national, district, subdistrict, or neighbourhood. It varies within various ENHR contexts. At the national level, the community may comprise national or international development NGOs, advocacy or pressure groups, support groups, television viewers, or readers of newspapers. At this level, *community* is often another term for civil society, the general public, or users of health services. At the district or subdistrict levels, the community may comprise local officials, health workers, grass-roots workers from large NGOs, community-based organizations, religious leaders, or a focus group drawn from various neighbourhoods in a district. At the neighbourhood level, planning and action may involve women who use certain water sources, members of a religious congregation, or residents of the catchment area of a health facility. Often community participation takes place at multiple levels.

Thinking about the levels of community participation raises the issue of representation. Who represents the community at a national priority-setting workshop or a village meeting? Who speaks and who is mute? In Bangladesh, officials from NGOs and various interest groups represent communities in the ENHR working group and national forum. In one view, such representation ensures community participation in the ENHR process; in another, "those are just politicians — they don't represent the people!" (see Box 4.5). There are no easy answers. All representation is partial, but it should be meaningful.

Box 4.5

NGOs and grass-roots representation in Bangladesh

With a population of about 123 million people and the vast majority of these living in rural areas, Bangladesh has faced a real problem of community representation. Nearly half of its citizens live in poverty, and only 45% of those who are 7 years of age and older are literate. The situation of women is of special concern. Local government structures are weak in terms of resources and development functions (UNDP 1996). In this setting, NGOs have played an enormous role — first in social-welfare activities and later in promoting community participation in development. It is said that Bangladesh is a country of NGOs. In the field of health and population alone, there are more than 2000 registered NGOs.

As noted in Box 4.1, BRAC was a key to establishing ENHR. In national workshops on ENHR, NGOs were well represented — in fact, they constituted the largest category of participants. Likewise, the national forum and the working group for ENHR have a weighty proportion of NGO representatives. The assumption seems to be that NGO involvement ensures community participation. But in what sense do NGOs represent communities?

The obvious answer is that NGOs are a community of interest, and they represent themselves in the ENHR process. But group discussions held in connection with the Bangladesh study suggested more concern with how the NGOs might represent their grass-roots target groups. One view was that there was indirect community participation in FNHR, because the NGO representatives belonged to organizations that work directly with the grass-roots-level people and therefore reflect their health needs and perspectives. A more critical view was that NGO executives are the ones who attend workshops and sit on committees; they have little direct interaction with poor village people. Lower level (frontline) NGO personnel might be better representatives.

Source: Choudhury (1999).

Tokenism can be found both in the selection of representatives and in the ways they participate. "Dragging community representatives along as proud exhibits of an inclusive process — without a genuine say — demeans the whole process of participation" (COHRED 1999, p. 2).

Commentators have said and written much about the importance of reaching the "real grass roots" and the "poorest of the poor." Indeed, this is critical to ENHR and equity-oriented development. The other two stakeholder groups have sometimes lost sight of the fact that ENHR inevitably challenges the priorities of traditional research communities; the politics of power is such that the voices of the poorest people, who bear the greatest burden of disease, are least audible. The other ENHR partners must, at the very least, ensure that they do not drown out those voices with their own.

The people whose work brings them into daily contact with marginalized groups are often, in practice, the ones who represent their interests to researchers and policymakers. It is important to determine whether the parties engaged in this activity are the best to reach the desired goals in a particular situation.

Organizations are one sort of party to speak for the marginalized or poorest of the poor. In a number of African countries, religious missions and NGOs working in health have traditionally played a strong role in providing improved access to health services to the poorest sections of the community. They, along with many other organizations, may be well poised to advocate equity in health on behalf of their clients or target groups (Jareg and Kaseje 1998).

Elected or appointed officials (in particular, middle- and lower level officials) may also be legitimate representatives and spokespeople for their communities. Even when there is doubt about this, it is usually advisable to try to include such officials. From one point of view, health workers are part of the communities in which they work and are well placed to represent the people and problems they confront every day; from another, they are themselves a community. One needs to remember that their interests may not be exactly the same as those of their patients, although they may have a good understanding of the health needs of the community.

Community workers recognize the importance of local opinion leaders. Opinion leaders not only speak for and represent the community but also exert power and influence — sometimes because they are wealthier, control important resources, or are more educated and articulate, but often because of personal qualities like moral authority, intelligence, or energy. Researchers sometimes see opinion leaders as a problem in community-based projects: one research project in Guinea excluded local leaders from focus-group discussions because they tended to dominate the discussion (Haddad et al. 1998). But another project in the same country emphasized how important it is to use local leaders as conduits for reaching the project target group (Sylla and Diallo 1999).

In many countries, women's voices are seldom heard in public gatherings. Men speak for the women. Where the men are more educated and have more time and better contacts with influential people, men are more likely than women to represent their community and participate in research in all the various ways that people can. This can be disadvantageous for women and impractical insofar as women's views are relevant to the problem under investigation. But there can also be a positive side to involving men more thoroughly in health issues, especially where researchers and policymakers have tended to see family health as the sole responsibility of mothers.

When researchers and policymakers address some people and not others as representatives of communities, they may strengthen existing forms of organization or help to create new ones. Addressing problems of inequity in health means asking whose voice is not being heard and striving to include it in health and development discussions. Without such voices, discussions of equity may be abstract and academic. Long-term field researchers or thoughtful service providers may be helpful in pointing out who would be likely to be silent. More importantly, one needs to create windows to view local realities from the national level: "Local experience provides a constant point of reference for monitoring the move toward equity, and should be firmly linked to national priority setting processes, resource allocation for research, and information dissemination" (COHRED 1999, p. 5). Establishing a strong ENHR portfolio of community-oriented research projects provides the widest of windows possible. In future, national research-coordinating mechanisms need to establish guidelines or a policy on the use of participatory methods of research or on encouraging community participation in ENHR projects. At present, few country ENHR mechanisms have set out criteria on community participation for use in evaluating projects.

WHEN IS COMMUNITY PARTICIPATION IN RESEARCH RELEVANT?

A distinction is often made between applied and basic research. The assumption is that community participation is mainly relevant to applied research. It is perhaps easiest for people to see some potential or relevance of research for their lives when the problems occur at the level of experience, such as accessing health services and feeding children, rather than at the level of microbiology or pharmacology. But here, too, researchers and policymakers need to show greater open-mindedness in deciding what community participation means (see Box 4.6).

> **Box 4.6**
>
> ### Another kind of community participation in Trinidad
>
> In Trinidad and Tobago, as in other member countries of the Caribbean Health Research Council, community participation has not been a central aspect of health research. In 337 papers presented at the regional scientific meetings over the last 3 years, none mentioned consultation with communities in the selection, design, or implementation of the research. But in that same period, a drama has been unfolding on the national stage that reminds us that community participation can take many forms.
>
> When the country was selected as a possible site for phase II HIV–AIDS-vaccine trials, external research collaborators gave a mandate to national researchers at the Medical Research Foundation to make preparations in the event the government gave its consent to proceed with the trials. What followed might be described as attempts to create a community.
>
> Trinidad and Tobago is a small country of 1.2 million people, with a well-developed media and communication sector. The possibility of the AIDS-vaccine trial provoked a lively debate in newspapers and on radio and television. A full-page advertisement against the trials was taken out in a national newspaper. The researchers soon realized that many people were not well informed about research, much less about AIDS-vaccine trials. The fear that thousands of Trinidadians would be used as guinea pigs was widespread. On television, people had learned about the syphilis research on black Americans in Tuskegee, and they realized that research can involve risk and humiliation. AIDS itself was a poorly understood and sometimes divisive issue. Some religious groups opposed any discussion of sexuality. The mandate to inform about the vaccine trials became the much larger task of communicating about the prevention and treatment of AIDS, the situation of people living with the disease, and the role of research in dealing with it.
>
> With the help of two community consultants and with support from an international network of researchers and AIDS advocacy groups, steps were taken to reach out to the public. A 1-day workshop was held for journalists. The staff of the national AIDS hotline, which was established early in the 1980s, were trained to respond to questions from the public concerning the proposed vaccine trial. The community consultants appeared on television over several months. There were meetings with professional organizations. Once the issue became widely known, the community consultants and researchers were invited to speak to groups like the Organization of Science Teachers. Most important, a Community Advisory Board (CAB) was established to advocate vaccine trials, inform the public, and act as a watchdog for the interests of the public and those who might eventually become research subjects. CAB consists of 20 people; most represent interested organizations; some are media consultants or people whose lives are touched by AIDS.
>
> *(continued)*

> **Box 4.6 concluded.**
>
> The process is ongoing. Even within CAB, consensus and respect for difference need to be built. The members have been getting training in how and what to communicate and planning how to go ahead. The Ministry of Health has established an Ethics Committee to review the scientific aspects, as well as ethical issues, of the proposed vaccine-trial protocol and advise the Ministry accordingly. Public opinion is still divided, and many people are not yet well informed. But what is important is that research has been brought to public attention. A community of interest has been established, even though the interests are often conflicting. An advocacy group is working to promote understanding of the nature of, and need for, research on AIDS. As one of those involved explained, "It is an educational process to get the community to the point of being able to make decisions about research and to see how research could help."
>
> Source: Francis and Picou (1999).

Operational studies and action research have tended to lend themselves best to community participation. They are as much about taking action to solve problems as doing research in the strict academic sense. Systematic attempts to find new ways to manage problems follow joint explorations of local conditions by community members and researchers. This kind of learning for a purpose makes sense to the research subjects.

Epidemiological and survey studies have been seen to offer little scope for community participation. Sometimes researchers train members of the community as enumerators. But beyond being dutiful respondents, community members are generally not involved. There are, however, exceptions that point to the need to reevaluate this view. Community Information, Empowerment, Transparency International, for example, has successfully involved community members as coresearchers in the conduct of sentinel community surveys, which combine qualitative and quantitative data from household questionnaires, reviews of institutional data, key-informant interviews, focus groups, and geographic information systems (Andersson 1996).

Whether on health economics or perceptions of diarrhea, social-science research is not necessarily operational research. In health-systems research, policy analysis, and community studies, researchers usually do the planning and data-gathering. The subjects of the research do not become coresearchers. (In fact, in ethnographic research, the idea is that the researcher participates in people's projects, rather than they in the researcher's.) Still, researchers can ask themselves whether their work is relevant to anyone outside of the academic community. Identifying an interested group and communicating research findings to create interest are also ways of creating a relationship with the third stakeholder in ENHR.

Basic or clinical research on specific diseases remains the most common type of health research in many countries. What kinds of community involvement, if any, can happen here? Lay people may help to collect biomedical data, and they may even take part in analyzing it. In a community-based malaria-intervention project in the Philippines, for example, lay people learned to identify and collect certain types of mosquitos and helped to collect and read blood smears (Batangan and Ujano-Batangan 1999). The Consumer Network of the Cochrane Collaboration affords an example of another avenue for community participation in clinical research (see Box 4.7).

Primary health-care workers, as a community, may also be an important group to communicate with about disease research. In Trinidad and Tobago, researchers worked with local health workers to develop treatment guidelines for common diseases. In some countries, advocacy and support groups are in place for people with chronic diseases or disabilities — HIV–AIDS, diabetes, heart disease. Involvement with such groups may also afford opportunities for community participation. Fundamentally, however, community participation rests on the relationship between researchers and communities and the expectations of each for the research process.

WHAT KINDS OF RELATIONS EXIST BETWEEN RESEARCHERS AND COMMUNITIES?

Community demand and the duration of research projects are the two most important dimensions of relationships between communities and researchers. Most health research is short term. Researchers working with a patient group or geopolitical unit are happy if they finish their data collection and analysis before their funding ends. Because the time frame is short, there is usually little reciprocity in this type of relationship. The researcher has no obligation to the community in the long run. Although communities can be involved, the researchers have limited opportunity for a continuing dialogue with subjects. Of course, researchers can use what they learn in a dialogue with another community. But most often, they feel they have met the ethical obligation to disseminate the results of their research when they report to their sponsors, colleagues, or perhaps a national institution.

Some research projects are embedded in a long-term relationship with a community (Das Gupta et al. 1997). This may be the case

> **Box 4.7**
>
> ### Consumer participation in better health decisions
>
> Health-care consumers and health professionals, particularly in developed countries, are currently swamped by the latest and sometimes conflicting research findings reported in health-care journals and relayed through the media. Sorting out the wheat from the chaff and staying up to date are critical but increasingly difficult tasks.
>
> The Cochrane Collaboration is an international effort by researchers, practitioners, and consumers to sift through health-care research, find as many controlled trials as possible, analyze them, and make this information as accessible as possible. The aim is to help people to make better decisions in health — whether they are practitioners, consumers, policymakers, or researchers.
>
> Consumers actively participate in many parts of the Cochrane Collaboration by helping to decide its directions, priorities, and products, as well as through being involved in the production of reviews and helping to spread the information more widely in their communities. Consumers help to define the full range of benefits and problems of health-care interventions, consider available evidence, and make recommendations for future research. Consumers are also involved in making these reviews easier to understand.
>
> The Consumer Network of the Cochrane Collaboration encourages consumer participation, helps consumers get in touch with each other, and produces information for them. This includes preparing quick- and easy-to-read minisynopses of all new Cochrane reviews, as well as tools such as a research glossary for consumers. Since 1999 the Consumer Network has worked to develop consumer participation in the Cochrane Collaboration from developing countries, with an emphasis on Africa. Involvement has grown steadily, with a plan for African consumers and community groups to actively shape health-care research and activities in the Cochrane Collaboration, their local communities, and internationally. A second focal point for developing-country consumers is the Reproductive Health Library, published jointly by the World Health Organization and the Cochrane Collaboration and made available free of charge. Consumers with an interest in reproductive health have formed an advisory group to advance consumer participation. Activities include participation in priority-setting, incorporation of material written by consumers in the library, and exploration of the potential for producing evidence-based health information for consumers in developing countries.
>
> For more information, visit the Network's website at http://hiru.mcmaster.ca/cochrane/cochrane/consumer.htm.

where research stations and community health training have been established. The International Network for Demographic Evaluation of Populations and Their Health, for example, brings together longitudinal research projects based at 20 field sites in sub-Saharan Africa (Tollman and Zwi 2000). A series of research projects may be linked to a long-term epidemiological study, with researchers following cohorts over many years. These sorts of research offer better opportunities for people to get to know about the research. They know where they can find the researchers again. Often these are the sites where people receive health-care services, so they associate the research with some kind of benefit to their community.

Communities do not usually spontaneously ask to become involved in research. It is a fundamental fact about the relationship between researchers and communities that researchers generally take the initiative. Communities — or the public in general — are seen as the ultimate beneficiaries of research, but not as immediate users who might actually request it (COHRED 2000e). Yet, this would happen more frequently if frameworks were in place to facilitate contacts and acquaint communities with the potential uses of research.

Development projects are probably the most important users of research in many countries. Where there is a high dependence on development assistance, the initiative to commission a study often comes from the funders. Occasionally, workers involved in local development efforts request technical support to carry out studies, as did those involved in the Pallisa Community Development Trust project in Uganda (Okurut et al. 1996). In either case, communities are users of research to the extent that they link the creation of knowledge to the solution of concrete problems.

A user orientation toward research has to be sensitive to community problems and interests, particularly areas in which specific groups might see a need for the research. Health workers may want to systematically gather information on a problem arising in the course of their work. Advocacy groups may be interested in research as a basis for legislative or administrative change. In South Africa, the Reproductive Rights Alliance presented research results to the Parliamentary Portfolio Committee on Health to support its argument for legislative change (see its website at http://www.healthlink.org.za/rra). In many countries, one sees a growing number of support or interest groups with a focus on particular diseases or conditions: people with AIDS or other chronic diseases, disabilities, or problems with alcohol or drugs. The Diabetes Association of Trinidad and Tobago had research topics it wanted studied; it knew that research had been done in their country on this priority health problem and wondered why no researcher had ever contacted it.

The issue of how researchers and communities relate to each other is partly a question of frameworks and institutions. It is not necessarily the case that one overall national coordinating body will have responsibility for fostering such relationships. Part of the task of an ENHR mechanism may be to identify frameworks to support contacts between the two parties and strengthen communities' capacities to use research results. Existing community health-research and training programs would be an obvious place to start. Such programs should be in place to prepare future health researchers "to encourage dialogue with local government and community leaders in developing community-based, partnership-driven research" (COHRED 1996, p. 33). Box 4.8 provides an example of a medical-school curriculum that incorporates training in participatory development. Other examples are the faculties of medicine at Suez Canal University, Egypt (Nooman and Mishriky 1991), University of Ilorin, Nigeria (Ogunbode 1991), and Chulalongkorn University, Thailand (Suwanwela 1991).

WHAT ARE THE EXPECTATIONS AND TRADE-OFFS OF COMMUNITY PARTICIPATION?

Although researchers and communities may share a long-term commitment to improving health — even to equity in health — in the short term they usually have divergent interests and expectations.

Box 4.8

University–community alliances in the Philippines

The Philippines has a long tradition of community organizing and development work, as well as a rich assortment of NGOs. From both flow positive attitudes and experiences about people's involvement in solving their own problems. There is also widespread acceptance that operational research should be a part of these efforts. Real dialogue takes time to develop and appreciation of the process needs to be instilled in future researchers as part of their training. To this end several medical schools have established programs in community participatory development.

One of these is the Zamboanga Medical School Foundation, which collaborates with the Pediatric Research Center for Mindanao, the Regional Health Office of the Department of Health, and the Local Government Units in Region 9. Medical students learn community-participation strategies in their problem-based medical curriculum. They are assigned to rural health units in underserved areas, and they have a commitment to working within an intersectoral framework for community participation, rather than just focusing on narrow medical issues. The goal is to develop participatory intervention programs for priority health problems.

This is a long-term alliance between a training institution and a geo-political community. Students rotate through, junior students overlapping with senior ones, to maintain continuity and avoid repetition.

Source: Batangan and Ujano-Batangan (1999).

Researchers see their work as one of creating new knowledge, and they feel they are only accountable to their colleagues and sponsors. For them, some degree of community participation generally facilitates the research in terms of compliance and logistics. Many appreciate the ways that community involvement poses challenging and socially relevant problems. But it also demands resources, especially time, to carry on a dialogue and attend to the interests of community members, which often conflict with those of the research. It is troublesome that community expectations do not correspond to research goals and methods. Researchers need to understand that this is not just an obstacle, but an issue deserving careful scholarly attention. Box 4.9 describes an NGO–community partnership built on the researchers' long-term engagement and sensitivity to the complex social and cultural dynamics of a community.

By and large, communities are less interested in knowledge for its own sake; they are concerned with its possible relevance to their lives. Countries show great differences in the extent to which members of the public understand the concept of academic research, even in a country like Trinidad and Tobago, where the level of education is reasonably high. Nevertheless, community members often have positive expectations (see Box 4.10). Initially, they may hope for material benefits and expect the government or the researchers to provide solutions to the problems under investigation. They desire to help themselves, their families, or others, and some have a genuine wish to gain new skills and knowledge. Insofar as researchers are significant outsiders or powerful elites (doctors, professors), community members may see an opportunity to gain influence through cooperation with them — at least, it is better not to be on their bad side.

Community members have trade-offs to make as well. The research makes demands on their time and material resources, often offering them no compensation. If their efforts seem to bear no fruit, they may feel bitter or lose interest. At worst, they may feel exploited. At the very least, they may feel that nothing came out of the research. They may not, for example, even hear anything about what the researchers found out. Although not all research projects can feed back results to their research subjects directly, one needs to recognize an issue of public accountability and communication that is too often neglected here.

In addition, some people have the simplistic view that researchers can identify the problems and expectations of communities once and for all. But those who have worked with communities emphasize that community participation develops over time; expectations change as communication develops.

Box 4.9

Lessons from an NGO–community partnership for women

The Panay Development Institute was formed in 1984 by a small group of academics and professionals, based in Metro Manila, who wanted to help communities become self-reliant. In 1987, the organization changed its name to the Panay Self-Reliance Institute (PANSRI). The commitment, determination, and skills of the fledgling NGO would be challenged in the years and projects ahead. In the community of Pangaraykay, it has learned the importance of long-term, highly engaged involvement with the people whom it hopes to empower.

Pangaraykay (the pseudonym chosen by the NGO to protect the community's identity) is a Hiligaynon word meaning to scratch the earth for food, persist, and be patient. It captures the essence not only of the community but also of the lessons learned by the NGO: hard work resulting in seemingly small changes, persistence, and patience.

In consultation with the Pangaraykay women leaders and friends in other NGOs, PANSRI formulated Project UPLIFT Pangaraykay (or Upland Program for Livelihood and Improvement of Farm Technology in Pangaraykay), funded by the Canadian International Development Agency. Led by the women of Pangaraykay, the project was an undertaking of the entire community to improve its economic self-sufficiency through a community-based seed bank, a rice mill, a cooperative store, adoption of technology for sustainable agriculture, and skills transfer.

Transcending fear of outsiders and NGOs was a first step that needed to be taken by this community, traumatized by militarization. Self-interest, jealousy, petty corruption, patriarchal traditions, and personal power struggles within the community threatened to collapse several of the initiatives shortly after they began. The PANSRI team gained sensitivity to the cultural and gender values against the open airing of grievances and criticisms and learned how to coax underlying issues to the surface of discussions. As well, they learned to swallow their own frustration and overcome the inclination to step in and fix problems for people.

The success of PANSRI's relationship with the community lies in a process of continuing negotiation. The villagers' insistence, for example, on the choice of a male leader of one initiative was against the goal of creating opportunities for female leadership. The NGO learned that it was necessary to be flexible in the short term, without compromising basic principles over the long term.

The road to empowerment has proven long and the journey arduous. Together, Pangaraykay and PANSRI have traversed the first few miles.

Source: Estandarte et al. (2000).

> **Box 4.10**
>
> **Community expectations in Guinea**
>
> Interviews with 160 residents of three rural areas concerning their experiences and views of community participation in research revealed that many people were unfamiliar with the concept of research itself. Almost two-thirds of the respondents said that no research had been done in their area. With the concept explained to them, the majority were able to express some expectations about their role and that of researchers. When informed and mobilized by local officials, residents indicated they would be ready to assist in answering questions, helping researchers, and providing food and lodging. They felt, however, that the resolution of their problems should be the responsibility of the researchers and the authorities. The community members wanted medicines and health facilities.
>
> A different pattern emerged in one of the localities studied, Kissidougou, where action research had been carried out in connection with the establishment of a health-insurance program. Partage de risques maladie (PRIMA) was a collaborative effort between local residents, the government, and the German development agency, Gesellschaft für Technische Zusammenarbeit (GTZ, agency for technical cooperation). GTZ had been working in the area and had financed a health centre. A German volunteer started a maternity centre. Although these were not strictly part of PRIMA, many people associated the action research, health-insurance scheme, and new facilities with this project. The concrete outcome was important. In contrast, respondents in areas where research had not brought any advantages expressed disappointment.
>
> The establishment of PRIMA was a process in which participatory-research methods were used to jointly explore health problems and resources. People who had been involved were more articulate about their health problems than respondents in the other localities. A climate of dialogue was established in which they learned to discuss, clarify their ideas, and reflect on their problems. Their view of community participation was correspondingly different. They expected researchers to define strategies together with them and to work together to put research into action.
>
> An important final point about community expectations in Guinea is that even though people wanted concrete benefits, they also wanted information and feedback on what the researchers had found out. They thought authorities should insist on researchers sharing their knowledge.
>
> Source: Sylla and Diallo (1999).

A FRESH PERSPECTIVE ON COMMUNITY PARTICIPATION IN ENHR

The experience of most countries with ENHR, to date, has been with the difficult work of promotion and advocacy, establishing an ENHR mechanism, creating or reshaping the national health-research agenda, and mobilizing financial support for the mechanism and the agenda. However, as the ENHR process matures and coordinating bodies for national health research settle into the core business of working toward equity in health and linking research to action (COHRED 2000e) they will clearly need to reframe third-stakeholder involvement in these goal-oriented terms, rather than in the activity-oriented terms of the original seven-element ENHR strategy. Specifically, it may be more fruitful to think about how communities can participate in linking research to action than about how they can become involved in promotion and advocacy or priority-setting. Both these strategic activities are about, for example, fostering ongoing dialogue among the various partners to link research to action.

COMMUNITY PARTICIPATION IN WORKING TOWARD EQUITY IN HEALTH

A first step in working toward equity in health will be to bring the dimensions of inequity to the attention of the public. Communication of research findings about health inequities will therefore be essential. But what kind of communication is most meaningful and to whom? Traditionally, epidemiological surveys have been powerful ways for advocates to garner support for views when presenting arguments to politicians — numbers are seen as facts. Yet, research with strong elements of community participation may be equally convincing, or even more effective in motivating change. Communication that incorporates the voices of marginalized or struggling people, especially if they are active agents looking for allies, gives a human dimension to the movement for equity. Journalists are experts at bringing out the personal touch of a pitiful case, but this is not what is needed. Rather, communication should show the dimensions of inequity as experienced and managed by a community of social actors.

Focusing on the involvement of marginalized groups in research can bring them more actively into the struggle for equity. It is not just a question of giving vulnerable groups opportunities to improve their health, but also one of supporting them in creating these opportunities. The problem is that often the most vulnerable people are least likely to participate. Creating equity means helping these people find allies in a community of action and advocacy — it also means empowering the communities, themselves, to define their health needs and seek solutions to them.

COMMUNITY PARTICIPATION IN LINKING RESEARCH TO ACTION FOR DEVELOPMENT

Linking research to action is often seen as the affair of researchers and policymakers. It is assumed that policy is the key to action and that research must feed into policy. The communities need to play a more active role in the process, and researchers and policymakers should not see them merely as "consumers" of research or targets of action.

Community participation can be a potent force for action in at least three ways:

— Community involvement encourages research for action, as communities are most interested in research relevant to the problems they experience. They want useful research, and they are particularly keen on operational research, in which the researchers implement and test new knowledge.

— An educated public or community can push policymakers to take action. Public pressure is important in democratic societies, even in undemocratic ones. When dissemination of research results creates awareness of health problems, inequities, and possible solutions, it can contribute to a momentum for change.

— Participation can empower people to act on their own behalf. To the extent that community involvement helps people to articulate their problems, to learn, acquire, and practice new skills, and to make allies, they are better able to be active and responsible. This does not mean that communities should solve their own health problems (the health and well-being of the citizenry is as much a responsibility of the state as of the individual, family, or community). However, it should be clear that people are not simply passive recipients of health services or wholly dependent on the knowledge of experts.

TOWARD LEARNING AND INNOVATIVE COALITIONS

Many researchers think that community participation is about listening to "the people" (or the organizations that purport to represent their interests). To truly make a difference in linking research to action and in working toward equity in health, the relationship between communities and the other stakeholders must be one of continuing dialogue. It is by reciprocal communication, not by one-way listening, that researchers, communities, and other partners can build coalitions. Such coalitions draw on the knowledge and experience of all partners to define common goals, acquire new understanding, and develop solutions to specific health problems. In this sense, learning and innovative coalitions reflect the newly emerging paradigm in health research (Pellegrini et al. 1998; Higginbotham et al. 2001) and knowledge production (Gibbons et al. 1994), in which "real-world problems" demand transdisciplinary perspectives and action. Learning and innovative coalitions defy single-discipline and single-stakeholder solutions. They recognize multiple sites of knowledge generation, many of which are outside of traditional institutions like universities (Harrison and Neufeld 2000). These coalitions require greater flexibility and a more long-term approach. Instead of thinking in terms of conventional individual research protocols with set objectives, researchers may have to think in terms of phases or a series of projects or a framework for continuing exchange.

Attempting to establish dialogue puts an obligation on researchers to communicate about their research in appropriate ways. Disseminating findings should be a part of ENHR. One possibility would be to make this a requirement of an ethical code, like informed consent or protection of research subjects. Another strategy would be to better equip researchers to perform this task by training them in some of the necessary communication skills. In many countries, collaboration with the media is the most common strategy. Workshops can be held for journalists, and they can be hired to help publicize research findings. Whatever strategy the researchers adopt, they should have channels to allow community members to express their views and ask questions. Where a project has access to the media and good communication infrastructure, it is possible to use radio call-in shows, telephone hotlines, and health-advice columns to answer community members' questions. Face-to-face communication would be the primary strategy in many settings, but a single dissemination workshop is not enough. Researchers need to meet communities in a variety of situations over time, so that they have real opportunities to learn to communicate.

ENHR is based on the principle that researchers are accountable to the society in which they work. Researchers should learn of and discuss this ethic when they are learning research skills. Putting medical students through a community medicine program is a start, but it is not sufficient. University curricula should include training on relationships between researchers, policymakers, and the public.

Future researchers should learn about the dilemmas of accountability (To whom? About what?) and about the various ways of relating to various kinds of communities.

Civil-society organizations may have special roles to play in coalition-building. They have an institutional character that persists over time and provides a framework. If they emphasize internal dialogue, as well as external communication between leaders and researchers, they can be genuine representatives in a coalition. Structures need to be in place to encourage relationships between organizations and researchers, and here policymakers can take steps to establish an organ or channel of communication.

One possibility is what is known in some North American and European countries as "science shops." They function as a link between universities and communities in larger society: noncommercial organizations define problems for research and contact the science shop, which in turn links graduate students and their supervisors with these potential users of research. In other words, the science shop recognizes communities as consumers of research and gives young researchers the opportunity for apprenticeships with organizations in need of their services. At the University of Copenhagen, the science-shop office is run by experienced students, who make contacts with all kinds of agencies, from patient organizations to sections of local government. They help students negotiate research projects and ensure that the results are disseminated to clients in useful ways.

In the past decade of ENHR, the ideal of collaboration among communities, policymakers, and researchers was phrased in terms of links between stakeholders. The term *stakeholder* suggests that a party has an interest in an enterprise, something to gain or lose. The term *iron triangle* of stakeholders (researchers, policymakers, and community) conveys a sense of rigidity, as if their interaction comprises a series of linear communications and trade-offs between the three groups. *Coalition* has another flavour. It is more action oriented, suggesting issue-based alliances, debates, and negotiation between disparate parties. Coalition members sometimes have conflicting interests, but commitment to a coalition implies an effort to accomplish something together, despite differences. In the next decade of health research for development, it may be most fruitful to think of community–researcher relations as coalitions for defining problems and learning to solve them.

CHAPTER 5

LINKING RESEARCH TO POLICY AND ACTION

Somsak Chunharas

SUMMARY

A key element in ensuring that health research indeed becomes an "essential link to equity in development" is creating a dynamic link between research and policy. In describing this challenge in 1990, the Commission on Health Research for Development outlined four pathways by which research can lead to health improvement: identifying and setting priorities, enhancing the efficiency and quality of health-care systems, developing new technologies and interventions, and advancing basic knowledge of human biology and behaviour.

This chapter analyzes some of the experiences of developing countries in strengthening this link over the past 10 years. It begins by identifying the key components of effective research–policy linkages. These include the dual processes of research and policy development, the context in which they both operate, the stakeholders involved, the products or outputs of both processes, and the critical role of mediators.

To begin, we must try to understand the attitudes of key stakeholders. Researchers typically feel they should remain "objective" in their work and are uncomfortable about close contacts with either decision-makers or the community. Decision-makers often regard researchers as too "academic," impractical, and slow, as the decision-makers work in an environment in which they must try to balance the demands of various pressure groups. Members of the community, an often forgotten stakeholder in the research process, may feel intimidated by both researchers and decision-makers, even though, given the opportunity, community members can have much to say about issues to investigate and the exact application of new knowledge.

Much more attention should focus on the social, political, and economic context of knowledge production and use. This principle is particularly important if the goal is to conduct and apply research relevant to a country's needs. At one level, science and technology (S&T) cannot thrive when a country is involved in armed conflict or has a dictatorial regime. Indeed, there are some sad examples in which the squelching of processes to nurture and apply science actually contributed to reversing gains in the health and welfare of people. At the more local level, people have sometimes refused to use the fruits of S&T because researchers failed to study and understand their deep-seated practices and traditions.

This chapter particularly emphasizes the importance of mediators in bridging the two parallel processes of research and policy development. It puts forward the proposal that various mediators can play distinctive and complementary roles in achieving successful linkages between research and action:

— Researchers themselves can develop some skills of communication and advocacy. In particular they must understand how decision-makers make resource-allocation decisions and how policymakers develop, implement, and monitor policies.

— This chapter makes a special plea for giving more attention to the critical role of national health-research managers, preferably within the context of an Essential National Health Research (ENHR) mechanism or system. These leaders can be the researchers themselves, research users, or funders. They require skills such as facilitating the process of multistakeholder priority-setting, building coalitions to work on specific problems, seizing opportunities ("entry points") to identify relevant research questions or ensure the use of available research, and nurturing future leadership for national health research and development (R&D). In particular, these leaders must learn to function as "knowledge managers" within the rapidly changing context of the global knowledge economy.

— National governments also have an important role to play in improving both the technical and human infrastructure for social communication. Governments set the political climate by listening and responding to people's concerns, conducting the affairs of government openly and transparently, and asking for evidence to support decision-making. Political leaders must also understand that investing in S&T, both for short- and longer term purposes, is an investment in enhancing the well-being of people.

— Finally, the international research community has a major responsibility to ensure stronger links between research and policy. International agencies should consider changing the ways in which they have traditionally operated, for example, by aligning agency agendas with those of recipient countries, providing funding support directly to a multistakeholder national research structure, rethinking the function of technical assistance as a condition for funding, making much more use of national consultants (who understand the local context), and using external experts only for carefully negotiated distinctive contributions.

RESEARCH TO IMPROVE HEALTH

A growing expectation of health research is that it contribute to enhancing human development. Ten years ago, the Commission proclaimed it an "essential link to equity in development" (CHRD 1990). The Commission purposely defined *health research* in broad terms as "the generation of new knowledge using the scientific method to identify and deal with health problems" (CHRD 1990, p. 13). Given such a definition, health research encompasses many disciplines and includes epidemiology, policy, social sciences, management research, biomedicine, and clinical research. This definition also takes account of the fact that health research may be an undertaking not only of trained scientists but also of governmental- and nongovernmental-agency staff, district health managers, and even communities themselves, as discussed in Chapter 4.

The Commission outlined four pathways for research to lead to action to improve health (see Figure 5.1), each entailing a range of research topics and disciplinary perspectives (COHRED 1994, p. 10):

— *Identifying and setting priorities* — The first pathway involves studies of the distribution of health and disease, as well as of health care. It demands a continuous process of gathering and analyzing data about communities, including people's perceptions of health and disease. These data can enable researchers to assess the major determinants of health and disease in various segments of the population; identify the biological, behavioural, social, economic, and environmental risk factors and vulnerable groups; monitor changes; project trends; and recognize and combat epidemics.

— *Enhancing the efficiency and quality of health-care systems* — This pathway includes research into the use of health services; efficiency and cost-effectiveness of health interventions; evaluation and selection of technologies; assessment of the effectiveness of various combinations of medical, social, and other nonmedical interventions; design and testing of alternative approaches to delivering health care and financing health services; and, in regard to equity, the search for new ways to improve services to vulnerable, poor, and disadvantaged people.

— *Developing new technologies and interventions* — The third research pathway for health improvement involves the search for new biomedical tools, such as drugs, vaccines, diagnostic tests, and environmental-control measures for biological, chemical, and physical hazards; discovery and development of tools for disease control that are safe, simple to use, acceptable to communities, and affordable; and development of social, educational, and other interventions relevant to improving health.

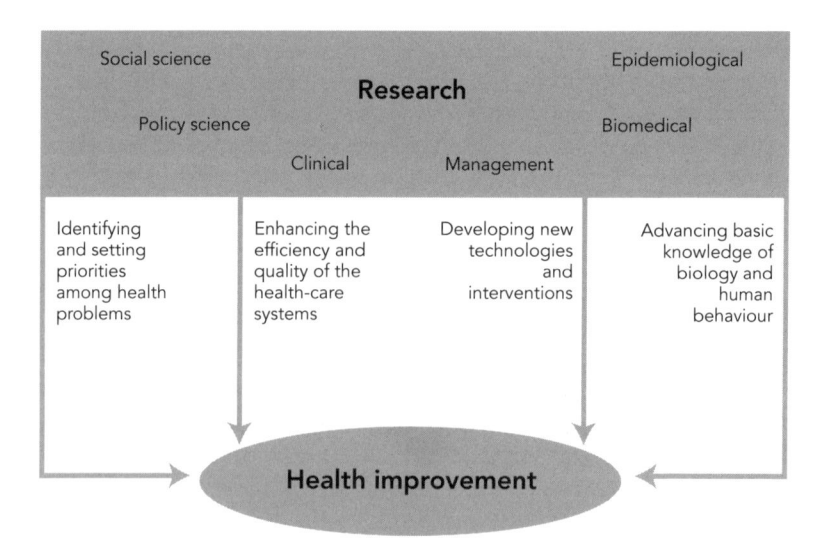

Figure 5.1. Pathways from research to health improvement.

— *Advancing basic knowledge of biology and human behaviour* — The final pathway includes achieving a better understanding of biological processes in health and disease; the biology of infective agents and their vectors; the role of genetic factors in resistance and susceptibility to disease; and advances in the understanding of health-related human behaviour.

A principal finding of the Commission, however, was that potential users of research (in particular, policymakers, health-care providers, and communities) tend to view research as peripheral to their interests and livelihoods. Moreover, much of the research being done, particularly in developing countries, is unrelated to local concerns and realities. The Task Force on Health Research for Development (TFHRD 1991) reported that a prevailing understanding within the research community is that policymakers often do not make use of research findings in decision-making. In addition, researchers feel that the managers of health-care programs are not always using research results or applying scientific methods in planning, monitoring, and evaluating the services they deliver. By the same token, policymakers, health-care managers, and the public have accused researchers of failing to address the health problems with top priority; moreover, the researchers often fail to make readily understandable and timely reports of their findings and recommendations to people outside the academic community. Some attribute this situation to a lack of effective interaction between researchers, policymakers, health-care providers, and communities and an absence of mediators to bridge the gap between research and action, specifically the gap between research and policy.

KEY COMPONENTS OF EFFECTIVE RESEARCH–POLICY LINKAGES

Strengthening the linkages between policy and research requires an understanding of the key components of their interface: the research and policy processes, stakeholders, mediators to help link the two processes, research products, and the larger context of decision-making and research. Walt (1994) and Trostle et al. (1999) described similar frameworks:

— *The research and policy processes* — It is important to pay attention to the research planning and execution and decision-making processes. We need to link many steps in both processes, not just the initial steps of defining research questions and policy priorities and later steps of disseminating results and implementing policies and programs. Linking the two processes may mean more than simply inviting policymakers to participate in research planning. It may be equally useful for researchers to participate in the policy- and program-development process, from which they can distil crucial research questions.

— *The stakeholders* — Decision-makers would be more likely to use research results if researchers identified the intended users (policymakers, donors, communities, or health-care providers) and involved them in formulating questions and problems.

— *Mediators* — Mediators are individuals or institutions with an active role in fostering linkages between the research and policy processes. They may be organizations supporting research work. They may be the researchers themselves. They may even be academic or civic groups supporting evidence-based decision-making. National research-coordinating bodies may also play a mediating role to better foster research-to-policy linkages. International agencies, too, have an important contribution to make as intermediaries in linking knowledge and action.

— *The products and outputs* — "Products" refers to the research studies themselves and how they link up to the decision-making process. In most cases, researchers are concerned about the quality of research as the criterion to determine whether to use it. The nature of the issues and the studies themselves, however, can also play a crucial role. Studies providing factual findings have a status and use different from those of studies with concrete recommendations and especially studies addressing a particular problem. In fact, it may be helpful to think of research products not as final reports at the end of research projects, but as a series of diverse outputs within an ongoing integrated program for both research and action. Sometimes researchers carry out several studies within a program and these lead to a single decision. In turn, experience with decisions and actions can lead to the next series of studies.

— *The context* — "Context" refers to the environment surrounding the research and decision-making processes. International organizations and existing funding structures have a significant impact on the linkage of research and policy, as do the socioeconomic and political situations of a country. Other important factors are the prevailing nature of the decision-making process and the influence of mass media.

With these components in mind, let us now look at developing-country experiences in linking research to policy, drawn from the Council on Health Research for Development's (COHRED's) Working Group on Research to Action and Policy (COHRED 2000f) and other available studies (Loewenson 1993; ADDR 1996). What lessons can we extract? What new ideas and actions might these sources suggest for addressing the research–policy gap?

DEVELOPING-COUNTRY EXPERIENCES IN LINKING RESEARCH TO POLICY

The most common approach to linking research to policy has been to produce good research and disseminate the results to the intended users. This relies on the assumption that decision-makers will always be receptive to relevant and useful information and make ready use of it once it is available. One cannot always make this assumption, as illustrated in some experiences from Burkina Faso (see Box 5.1). The success of such a supply-driven, linear approach hinges on ensuring that the intended users properly understand the research results. Consequently, a great deal of effort has gone into making the presentation of the research interesting and understandable. In fact, training courses and materials have been available to help researchers communicate more effectively (Porter 1995; SARA 1997). However, too often the emphasis has been on forging links with users once researchers have obtained the results, and not earlier in the process.

Over the last 10 years, more than 50 developing countries have adopted the ENHR strategy to support action promoting equity in health. Although various countries have adopted a variety of mechanisms to implement the ENHR strategy (COHRED 1999), all these mechanisms include an element of linkage between research and policymaking. Listed below are examples of the ways some countries have integrated ENHR into their social-development plans:

— In the Philippines, an autonomous ENHR Foundation works closely with the ENHR unit in the Ministry of Health to integrate the strategy into the National Health Plan. A detailed

> **Box 5.1**
>
> ### Researcher-driven policy development in Burkina Faso
>
> In rural Burkina Faso, child morbidity and mortality are extremely high, the quality and the use of the existing services are low while costs for treatment are out of reach, especially for the most vulnerable groups. Compelled by the findings from a series of studies on health services, medical care at the household level, and interhousehold distribution of disease, a group of researchers at the University of Heidelberg attempted to put the concept of *shared care* on the national health-policy agenda. The researchers saw themselves as advocates of a shared-care strategy and actively sought to communicate with, and involve, officials from the Ministry of Health (MOH) in the development of an intervention study in which mothers would be trained by village-health-centre staff to diagnose and treat common child diseases, as well as identify situations in which referral to professional health services is needed. Research results were disseminated in the form of reports and presentations to MOH officials and district physicians. In 1988, the concept of shared care was the topic of a workshop organized jointly by MOH and the University of Heidelberg.
>
> Despite the researchers' efforts, shared care has not been taken up by decision-makers. Absent was a sense of institutional ownership by MOH of either the research underlying the shared-care concept or the proposal for the intervention study. Indeed, there was general agreement among MOH officials that the issue of shared care had been put on the agenda by the researchers. One individual commented, "We asked ourselves whether these ideas had been parachuted from Heidelberg."
>
> Although MOH officials did not question the validity of the researchers' findings, they felt that a clearly defined strategy on how to proceed in the field was lacking. They also commented on the lack of mechanisms for monitoring and evaluation of the intervention. In addition, they perceived that their concerns in this regard received insufficient attention from the researchers.
>
> Another factor contributing to the failed uptake of shared care was that it was in competition with the recently established village-health-worker approach and did not fit into any of the major programs launched internationally.
>
> Researchers might have been more successful in putting shared care on the agenda if (1) greater ownership of the strategy had been encouraged by more actively involving decision-makers in the early stages of the research process; (2) efforts were made to embed the policy in the existing context by framing shared care as compatible with decentralization, cost control, and enhanced quality of care; and (3) communication was more two way, with stakeholders expressing their concerns and needs.
>
> Source: Gerhardus et al. (2000).

5-year research plan coincides with the research needs of this plan.

— In Kenya, the National Development Plan of 1994 incorporated a Master Plan of ENHR activities (1992–98). Kenya's priorities relate to maternal and child health, water and sanitation, health-care delivery systems, AIDS, and sexually transmitted diseases.

— In Ethiopia, a clearly articulated policy on science and development serves as a springboard for detailed policies and action plans for various economic and service sectors, and ENHR has a recognized role as an appropriate integrated strategy for organizing and managing research for health development.

— In Thailand, national development plans have formed the backbone of transformation and development for the past 36 years. Its 7th National Development Plan (1991–96) formally incorporates the ENHR strategy.

— In Jamaica, an ENHR Task Force has been active since 1995. Formally recognized by the Ministry of Health, it brings together representatives from the ministry, university-based units, and the Planning Institute of Jamaica in promoting and advocating ENHR.

— In Benin, a number of institutions have taken leadership in promoting ENHR. These include the Faculty of Health Sciences, the Regional Centre for Health and Population Development, and the Ministry of Public Health. ENHR also has a decentralized role within the Ministry and other organizations to allow for greater community participation. The strength of this arrangement has been the high level of participation from diverse interest groups. Its weaknesses have been its ill-defined interaction and lack of coordination with the Ministry of Public Health.

The experiences of these and others countries demonstrate that ENHR is making progress at the national level in linking research to action and policy. However, progress has been slow and uneven for a variety of reasons, including entrenched attitudes, ineffective communication strategies, and weak national funding arrangements. At another level, the sociopolitical realities of some countries or parts of countries prevent their establishing effective links between research and policy. In addition, international organizations involved in health research have a significant influence on what happens within a recipient country. Some aspects of these various challenges are explored below.

STAKEHOLDER ATTITUDES

Although many potential users of research results each have a role and contribution to make in linking research to action, most people have seen researchers and decision-makers alone as vital to increasing the probability of success and have largely ignored or overlooked the role of the community, the third stakeholder in ENHR. The values and attitudes of each of the three stakeholders bear further examination, as they can remove or create barriers in linking research to action.

RESEARCHERS

For the most part, researchers adhere to the idea that they should be unbiased and neutral with respect to the issues they study. With this attitude, they may resist "interference" from both decision-makers and the community. As a result, they may be reluctant to communicate with decision-makers during the research process and may be critical of information and suggestions from decision-makers or their staff. They may also have negative attitudes toward community involvement in the research process, viewing community members primarily as beneficiaries of the research. The researchers may believe that community members have too little information to make sound judgments about health priorities and problems and that sensationalistic and alarmist reports in the media sway their opinions. Some researchers may want to involve the community but are unsure of how to include them in the research process.

Despite a demonstrable demand for research to guide action, academicians often show a lack of capacity and interest in action-based research. This is partly due to the belief that research aimed at new discoveries or a better understanding of the natural world or human nature are of greater academic merit than that designed to guide decision-making. The latter type of research also tends to have short funding time frames. It may acquire the label "case-study research" because it deals with specific country situations, and for this reason international journals refuse to publish it. Such research is perceived to contribute little new knowledge to the global knowledge base. Such beliefs and practices discourage academicians from doing research for action. Without respect and acceptance from the academic community, studies to guide decision-making may fail to influence people in decision-making circles. Although the values described above are not universal and they are changing in some countries and institutions, many people undeniably still hold them, even in developing countries.

DECISION-MAKERS

Just as researchers may be sceptical of decision-makers and communities, decision-makers can have the same attitude toward researchers. Many decision-makers feel that researchers are too academic and theoretical. They see their recommendations as overly ideal or impractical. Researchers, they argue, fail to understand the reality of the health problems because they are, in many cases, distant from them. As a result of this attitude, decision-makers show a lack of interest in what researchers have to say about issues.

Politicians deal with demands from pressure groups and tend to respond more to the ideas and suggestions from these groups than to those of researchers. They may ignore evidence that fails to support these demands or accord it lesser priority. Consequently, such evidence may carry little weight unless it is acceptable to other societal groups with influence on decision-makers, whether they are politicians or administrators. We may have difficulty amending this attitude, and researchers need to understand it better if they want decision-makers to give proper attention to research findings. Researchers, in fact, may want to strengthen their own alliances with communities and those nongovernmental organizations (NGOs), forums, and groups acting in their interest. To better understand the realities confronting policymakers, researchers may find it helpful to invite thoughtful individuals to present their views about the linkage challenge (see Box 5.2).

THE COMMUNITY

The community, or the public in general, is an important stakeholder but is largely ignored in both decision-making and research. Researchers most commonly involve the community through participatory research, in which community members help to identify and seek solutions to local health problems. The community, however, can also be a crucial partner in determining the use of research for decisions and actions taken outside the community; researchers who wish to influence decision-makers through research should try to

> Box 5.2
>
> ## Using research findings: a policymaker's perspective
>
> How can research influence health policy? To help answer this question the International Health Policy Program invited three distinguished policymakers, including Mr Rajiv Misra, Secretary of Health in India from 1991 to 1994, to identify examples of research that had an impact on policy and to reflect on the sorts of factors that influence the use of research findings.
>
> In Mr Misra's experience, the kinds of research initiatives most likely to shape health policy and programs are those undertaken by the Ministry of Health.
>
> The impetus for such research is often a desire to delineate the extent and nature of a health problem or review a program's effectiveness. Such was the case with respect to India's National Programme for Control of Blindness (NPCB).
>
> A national blindness survey, lead by the ophthalmic adviser to the government, produced startling results and confirmed the impression that NPCB was making little impact. The prevalence of blindness was found to have increased from 1.38% in 1974 to 1.49% in 1985, despite the control program. It also revealed that the leading cause of blindness was no longer trachoma, but cataracts. In addition, the survey's findings highlighted the impact of demographic and epidemiological transitions, about which there was little awareness at the time. With this new information in hand, the government commissioned an evaluation of NPCB's operations to pinpoint its strengths and weaknesses and make recommendations to improve the program's cost-effectiveness and technical efficiency.
>
> Mr Misra observed that the mechanisms for bringing research results to the attention of policymakers are often inadequate. In this connection, "the quality of leadership within the Ministry of Health and its receptivity to research outcomes is vital" (Misra 1996, p. 25). The occurrence of an epidemic (such as AIDS or malaria) that garners a lot of media attention can bring research findings to policymakers' attention that would otherwise remain sitting on a shelf. Similarly, endorsement of a study and its findings by an international donor agency makes a qualitative difference in the attention it receives.
>
> Lastly, Mr Misra found that serious shortages of resources do not seem to impede any worthwhile research efforts: "... where policymakers are convinced that a need exists, funds have always been found, either by the Ministry of Health itself, or through the funds available in the WHO's [World Health Organization's] country budget, apart from the resources available through donor agencies" (Misra 1996, p. 26).
>
> Source: Misra (1996).

involve the community as much as possible, even if the political situation in a country does not yet allow it to get involved in the policy process. (A more detailed analysis of the role of the community as a participant in research can be found in Chapter 4.)

One of the difficulties of involving the community in research for action is that its participation is necessarily partial, particularly at the national and district levels. Researchers tend therefore to work with NGOs or civil-society groups representing the interests of communities. They may also work with officially appointed leaders of communities, sometimes overlooking the unofficial leaders. In urban settings, where people congregate more within their work environment than within their neighbourhoods, researchers may have difficulty identifying groups representative of community interests. Commonly, community members are "consulted" about their health needs and problems. They are seldom allowed to play an active role in decision-making processes.

COMMUNICATING RESEARCH RESULTS

An important aspect of linking research to policy is effective communication. This requires an effective communicator and means of communication. Various communication channels are already available. Researchers have created some specifically to convey messages about their health research to intended users. Others include the press, radio, television, and even the Internet. Communication channels may be both part of the process of conveying a message and the "context" that determines the ways policymakers link research to policy. A common communication channel is the technical workshop, where researchers present their findings. Experience has shown, however, that the decision-makers themselves seldom attend such workshops, as they are too busy; instead, they send their representatives, who may fail, however, to bring the message back to the decision-makers. And in many instances, the only people who attend the workshops are other academics interested in some technical aspect of the research.

Many institutions doing research to guide action invest a lot of their financial and human resources in effectively communicating their results to decision-makers. In addition to using the sorts of workshops or meetings already described, they often create various types of succinct, easy-to-read publications, with no technical jargon or complex figures and data. The International Health Policy Program (IHPP) is well known for advocating effective communication between researchers and decision-makers. It makes resources available not only for doing research but also for communicating its findings, primarily through dissemination workshops. Another example comes from the experience of the Health Systems Trust (HST) in South Africa, which evaluated the effectiveness of various communication strategies in getting messages across to decision-makers and influencing their decisions.

Often researchers and research communities create channels for communicating with decision-makers that allow the researchers to retain a neutral stance and not appear to be advocates of a particular issue or solution. However, the overall system and culture of communication within a country can directly or indirectly affect these channels of communication; researchers attempting to communicate evidence for decision-making may fare badly in countries where no one welcomes such an endeavour or no one takes it seriously. Even if the researchers would like to go beyond the accustomed dissemination workshop, they may find themselves without good supporting partners or infrastructure to increase their chances of making the research known. Publishers who can produce attractive print materials might be scarce. People who can make technical research easy to understand for various audiences might also be in short supply. A country's rules and regulations may constrain the mass media, or an invisible power may even threaten the media to make it stay away from such functions. Taken for granted in some societies, communication between people of diverse levels of power is not the norm in others. Again, in many countries, people still perceive it as too costly to purchase the infrastructure to support communication and dissemination of information. Added to this is a lack of appropriately skilled human resources in social communication, as opposed to commercial communication, which may be less difficult to find nowadays.

RESEARCH FUNDING

From a research-to-action point of view, funding for research plays an important role in determining the extent of the linkage between the research and decision-making processes. Some research-funding agencies play crucial roles in mediating between these processes, especially influential external donors, such as international banks that also provide development loans.

Even when research funds derive from national sources and the demand for research leading to action is high, countries do not always make financial resources readily available for such studies. In some countries with national sources of funds for research, the emphasis has still been on technology development; this was illustrated in Brazil (see Box 5.3). Although research leading to workable

> Box 5.3
>
> ### Vaccine development and production in Brazil
>
> Until the end of the 1970s, Brazil's vaccination needs, like those of many developing countries, were met by importing private production. In the early 1980s, when the demand for vaccines expanded (as a result of the success of the National Immunization Program [Programa Nacional de Imunizações]), and the National Health Quality Control Institute (Instituto Nacional de Controle de Qualidade em Saúde) was established, it became evident that domestic production capacity was inadequate and that locally produced vaccines were of poor quality. In response to the new health-policy requisites, private-sector laboratories stopped producing, precipitating a crisis in the supply of serums and vaccines.
>
> The Immunobiologicals Self-Sufficiency Program (ISSP, Programa de Autosuficiência en Imunobiológicos) was created in 1986, with a view to encouraging national production by a group of public institutions (primarily the Oswaldo Cruz Foundation and the Butantan Institute). Between 1986 and 1998, the Brazilian government invested some 150 million USD in the production capacity and quality of these two institutions.
>
> In contrast, there has been no significant source of funding for basic and applied research in vaccine development. Ministry of Health support for studies and research has been restricted solely to activities connected with short-term operational issues, such as conducting inquiries into vaccine coverage, evaluating the potency of various formulations and the corresponding level of serological response, surveys of adverse events, evaluation of the cold chain, and studies of health workers' training in syringe-handling.
>
> More surprising still is the fact that even the support given by ISSP specifically for production involved no funding for vaccine development, except for the hepatitis-B vaccine. Technological development — which must necessarily be built on a broad, complex research base — was secondary to obtaining operational production technology. As a consequence of this thinking, investment was concentrated in building work and equipment, whereas investment in research and development (R&D) and in highly skilled human-resource capacity-building took a back seat. Thus, from a science and technology point of view, there was great fragmentation and dispersion of efforts, which led to a lack of strategic focus, an accentuated academic-research slant, and insufficient emphasis on industrial absorption of research results. On the health-policy side, R&D activities were simply ignored as essential components of a national vaccine strategy.
>
> The lesson is that researchers and policy developers must work together to create an integrated problem-oriented program that incorporates the various kinds of research needed to meet a national goal.
>
> Source: Gadelha (2000).

technologies is highly desirable, especially when it results in large-scale manufacturing for either the domestic or the international market, it seems that most funding sources have given a much lower priority to research more directly aimed at guiding action.

In many countries, national research funds flow through agencies for S&T, where health research competes with research in other sectors, such as agriculture. Countries with a separate funding mechanism for health research may put an emphasis on technology development or use, paying little attention to policy decisions or program development. Developing countries need to strike a balance in health-research funding, based on their health priorities and their actual and potential research capabilities.

THE SOCIOPOLITICAL CONTEXT

Although a great deal of attention goes to strengthening the various components mentioned above, the overall context or environment seems to play a crucial, if not deciding, role in the linkage between research and policy. One would be naive to assume that overall societal values and practices will be supportive of the search for, and the use of, evidence, even despite the logical expectation that good evidence makes for good decisions. It would also be naive, however, to assume that evidence has no place or will have difficulty finding its place in societies less supportive of evidence- or knowledge-based decision-making. This depends on the extent to which societies see researchers and research communities as sources of solid evidence and reliable information. In a country where a dictatorial regime has dominated for a long time, it may not matter much how much evidence is available for a given decision; a story from Uruguay illustrates this unfortunate lesson (see Box 5.4). The other extreme is the theoretically ideal situation in which decision-makers consult researchers and all available evidence before making a decision. In most countries, the reality is somewhere between these two extremes. The public expects decision-makers to make use of good information to guide their decisions, rather than relying solely on their personal opinions or experiences. Decision-makers will make use of the various available sources of information to the extent they feel the pressure to do so. It is encouraging to note that in many countries the research communities are striving to create evidence- or knowledge-based societies. The situation is changing quickly, and it will be important in this dynamic global environment to provide opportunities for intercountry dialogue to share experiences and ideas.

> **Box 5.4**
>
> **Political upheaval in Uruguay and Chagas disease control**
>
> At times, the political circumstances within a country may not just be at odds with the notion of dialogue between stakeholders (in particular, researchers and decision-makers) but may result in the suppression of research and researchers by government powers. Uruguay offers a case in point.
>
> During the military dictatorship (1973–84), many of the country's cultural, social, political, and democratic structures were destroyed. Numerous scientists were either imprisoned or exiled, and the budget of the county's single university was drastically reduced, effectively dismantling teaching and research capacity and creating a deficit from which the country has not yet fully recovered.
>
> Several decades of extensive research, for example, had informed the design and implementation of a Chagas disease-control program in 1972 by the Hygiene Division of the Ministry of Health. The coup d'état 1 year later, however, subverted all national health priorities and removed many national and local authorities, putting the program in jeopardy. What followed was 10 years of poor program performance, in which there was a lack epidemiological surveillance and weak definition of entomological indices needed for supervision, assessment, and follow-up.
>
> It has taken another decade to rebuild the control program, as well as internal research capacity, links between researchers and decision-makers, and cooperation with external agencies and foreign research centres.
>
> Source: Salvatella, R.; Muzio, D.; Sánchez, D. 2000. Research to policy: the case of foot and mouth and Chagas disease eradication in Uruguay. Report prepared for COHRED's Working Group on Research to Policy. Unpublished report.

In countries where democracy or people-based politics is developing or gradually evolving, the place for evidence generation and dissemination is becoming more apparent. Researchers may find it easier to do their job. They may change their research strategies completely so that decision-makers properly know and use their results. It is in countries that still concentrate power in the hands of a few people or groups that researchers find it difficult to properly and effectively carry out their roles. They may even face problems in the initial stage of conceptualizing and planning a research study, not just after they have completed the research and are making efforts to disseminate their results.

THE INFLUENCE OF INTERNATIONAL ORGANIZATIONS FOR HEALTH RESEARCH

International organizations play a very important role in influencing health research in most developing countries, where research funds are scarce. They include not only those working specifically to support health research, but also those dealing with health development or even socioeconomic development in general. Research is as an entry point for these organizations to exert their influence on the direction of national health development or health in the context of socioeconomic-development policies. This can have either a positive or a negative outcome, depending on how the process unfolds and the nature of the relationship between those involved in the process.

A common criticism is that international organizations only support the research that fits their own agendas. Sometimes those agendas are relevant and useful for countries; at other times, they are at odds with national health-research priorities. Some countries have tried to address national priorities, but with the use of external expertise and little involvement of their own national counterparts. Even when these undertakings involve nationals, these people tend to have the role of assistants, rather than of researchers. Lack of equal partnership and lack of concern for a country's own context and needs still predominate. Those imposing "external" agendas may worsen the situation in a developing country by insisting on the use of external experts to carry out research studies rather than actively involving nationals in the undertaking. Use of external experts is often a condition on receiving loans from the major development banks for health- and social-sector reforms. Some international organizations even carry out studies without involving national researchers at all; they simply "inform" countries of their health-development situation and recommend strategies for addressing it. Walt et al. (1999a) and Buse (1999) have recently described and analyzed this unhealthy asymmetrical power relationship between donor agencies and recipient countries and made suggestions on ways to change the attitudes and behaviours of both recipients and donors.

Having to rely on external sources of funding and follow externally imposed research agendas are common problems facing most developing countries. Such factors need not always lead to difficulties in creating relevant research and effectively linking it to action. This depends on the ways international organizations work with a country's decision-makers and researchers. In some cases, external sources of funding for research have played a crucial role, not only in allowing countries to set their own priorities and conduct relevant research, but also in strengthening national expertise and capability. In addition to supporting specific research studies, IHPP has provided funding for research dissemination and capacity-building consistent with national priorities. The Rockefeller Foundation initiated National Epidemiology Boards in Cameroon, Mexico, and Thailand to assist these countries in health-situation analysis; this in turn contributed to their identifying national health-research priorities. The Kaiser Family Foundation supported HST in South Africa in more or less the same manner.

Most international health-research agencies, however, still adhere to the conventional style of work. They believe that by setting a global or regional research agenda they will help to better guide a developing country's health R&D. They also hold that good national researchers are scarce and that international experts are the best people to carry out the research crucial to policy development. They prefer to develop specific research programs and let countries compete for funds within those programs, rather than providing funds directly to countries to support research with high national priority. International organizations need to reconsider capacity-strengthening strategies to ensure that training grants match national health priorities. Capacity-strengthening support should go beyond individuals and institutions and include national networks and annual meetings. With such a broadened support, national groups doing research may contribute to action on a more sustainable basis, as opposed to contributing to it in an ad hoc manner reflecting the demands of external donors.

STRENGTHENING THE LINKAGE BETWEEN RESEARCH AND POLICY

Although good-quality research on policy-relevant issues, with well-packaged and well-targeted products, may succeed in informing decision-making processes, there is a pressing need to build sustainable linkages between research and policy to achieve development goals. To understand the factors contributing to a sustainable arrangement, researchers may find it useful to conduct detailed descriptive studies of the research-to-policy process (see Box 5.5).

Figure 5.2 presents a framework for addressing the research–policy gap. The framework incorporates the key components outlined earlier in this chapter; the research and policy processes are discrete but parallel, and dialogue among the various stakeholders links

> **Box 5.5**
>
> ## Health research and policy Links in Mexico: lessons from five case studies
>
> While the links between research and policy in the United States and Western Europe are well-researched, there are few descriptive studies of the relationship between health research and policy from developing countries. In a recent article in *Health Policy and Planning*, Trostle, Bronfman, and Langer reported the results of such a study from Mexico. The authors analyzed responses from interviews with researchers and policymakers associated with four vertical programs of the Mexican Ministry of Health (family planning, AIDS, immunization, and cholera).
>
> Identified were a number of factors related to content, actors, process, and context that enable or impede the uptake of research results:
>
> ### Content
>
> *Enabling factors*
>
> — Reputation of the researcher (as a proxy for quality of the research);
> — Type of research (biomedical research carries more weight than social-science research); and
> — Research that targets specific issues and offers short-term, concrete, and applicable results.
>
> *Impeding factors*
>
> — Researchers and policymakers "speak different languages";
> — Both want to own the process; and
> — "Mutual intellectual disdain."
>
> ### Actors
>
> *Enabling factors*
>
> — Bodies exist to establish priority health concerns and set a national health-research agenda;
> — Financial and normative support for research from international organizations; and
> — Supportive environments created by national research organizations.
>
> *Impeding factors*
>
> — Lack of technical background among decision-makers and media;
> — Sense that decision-makers value experience over evidence; and
> — Agendas of private industry and special-interest groups override the importance of research.
>
> *(continued)*

> Box 5.5 concluded.
>
> **Process**
>
> *Enabling factors*
> - Informal personal communication between researchers and policymakers;
> - Suggested solutions do not conflict with program operation and feasibility; and
> - Development and use of formal communication channels.
>
> *Impeding factors*
> - Narrow professional interests of researchers and policymakers.
>
> **Context**
>
> *Enabling factors*
> - Political and economic stability;
> - Appointment of researchers to decision-making positions; and
> - Urgency of the health problem.
>
> *Impeding factors*
> - Centralization of power and information;
> - Constant changeover of personnel at the administrative level; and
> - Restrictions on economic resources.
>
> Source: Trostle et al. (1999).

these processes at multiple stages. Stakeholders include many groups with diverse possible contributions to the various stages of the two processes, and these processes must properly involve them all. Many are potential mediators, including the researchers themselves, national health-research managers, governments, and the international research community. Each group can make a distinctive contribution to bridging the gap by fostering new ways of thinking, improving infrastructure, and introducing new practices. All the actions of mediators require sensitivity to the broader sociopolitical context. Lastly, the research products themselves need not be a single final output at the end of the research process but may be a series of outputs of a variety of types that occur throughout the research process and inform the next steps in the decision-making process. The remainder of this section focuses on the various mediators and their ability to act as catalysts in creating and sustaining effective linkages between research and policy.

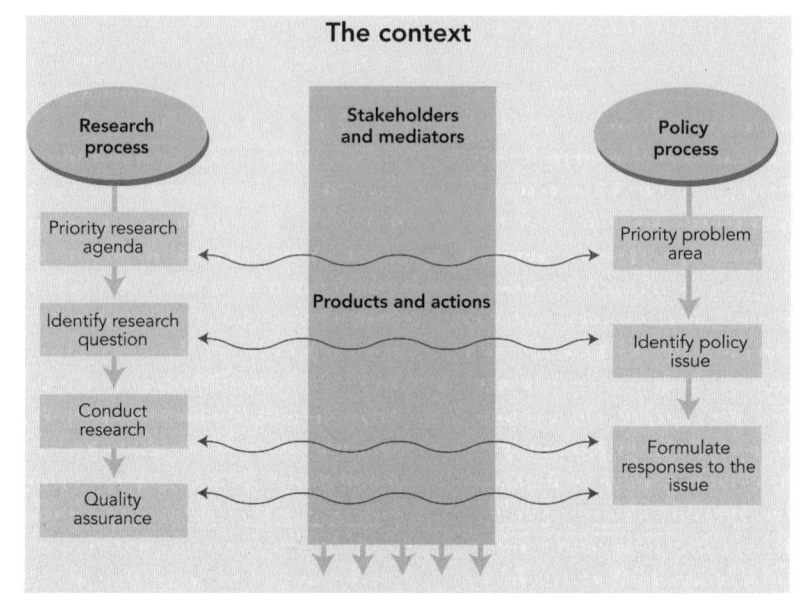

Figure 5.2. Strengthening research-to-policy linkages.

AN EXPANDED ROLE FOR RESEARCHERS

For researchers to have a place in the decision-making process, it is important that they not isolate themselves from it or allow decision-makers to deter them from participating in it. If research is to become an integral part of the decision-making process, then so too must researchers. This means that researchers must be involved in policy development or decision-making and not limit themselves solely to executing research. They may start their work by identifying research questions, based on a literature review or some theoretical conceptualization of interest to the academic community. But to make their research relevant to a decision-making process, they must become aware of the decision-making mechanisms and priority issues and concerns.

Researchers need to understand these issues from the perspective of the various stakeholders and take these points of view into account in formulating their research questions. However, they should not carry their solicitude for stakeholders and decision-makers so far that they compromise their objectivity or feel they need to obtain consent or endorsement from decision-makers.

Being involved in the decision-making process goes beyond the initial steps of identifying and formulating research questions. It also means that researchers have to be concerned about two parallel processes: one is the research process, in which the researchers are fully accountable for carrying out the best work possible; and the other is the decision-making process, which decision-makers may determine in response to their policy environment. Researchers will have to keep in mind the dynamics and progression of both processes and try to link them as they unfold. Researchers will, for example, need to consult periodically with the various stakeholders to ensure the relevance of the content, as well as the proper tempo, of the research work. This requires researchers to be fully aware of the context of the decision-making process and to interact with stakeholders and users of the research as much as possible, rather than carrying out their research in isolation and assuming that in the end good-quality research products will sell themselves.

Included among the various stakeholders and users of research are what one may broadly refer to as "the affected population," decision-makers, and intermediaries such as policy advisers, the media, and academics. Researchers need to recognize that actions resulting from their research affect many people. Such actions, therefore, often require the direct or indirect consent and cooperation of many other groups beyond the decision-makers. Working with those who can help to translate the messages into languages appropriate to the various groups of stakeholders therefore provides another entry point into the decision-making process. In this respect, researchers need to realize that they will have to work with many other groups beyond their academic peers. Some researchers are realizing that they can be both scientists and advocates, without compromising their scientific integrity (Brown 2000).

Researchers need to learn how to interact with these various groups of people. They must be prepared to listen to diverse viewpoints and perspectives. But more importantly, they must be able to incorporate them into their research, without sacrificing objectivity or neutrality. However, they must also be ready to communicate their ideas at various stages in the research process, as the decision making process demands. They cannot just be passive observers or participants in the decision-making process, afraid of losing their impartiality once they speak out. Being actively and properly engaged in the dialogue helps researchers understand how to incorporate various concerns and viewpoints into their research and identify the people who might be receptive to the research products.

Researchers strive to produce work of the highest scientific quality, and many feel that the products of their research will speak for themselves. An important way of letting research products do so is to publish them in academic journals, where researchers working in related fields will search eagerly for relevant new findings. Yet, researchers cannot afford to limit communication of their results to other members of the research community. Communicating with the larger public and policymakers is an essential part of being a good scientist, just as a surgeon's ability to communicate with patients is a crucial, but sometimes neglected, part of being a good surgeon.

The intended users of research constitute a broad group, and the ways and means of reaching them are quite different from those already familiar to researchers. Consequently, they need to learn new skills and adopt new attitudes to carry out their duties as social marketers. Social marketing involves getting the crucial messages across to the target population. It demands an ability to understand the target population in terms of its preferences and its style of learning new information so as to present the intended messages effectively.

Using marketing principles to disseminate research products means giving careful attention to packaging these products to make them attractive to various audiences. Timing is also important. Researchers need to be alert to opportune moments to present their results. Research marketing involves teamwork and requires the help of nonresearch professionals to formulate difficult technical messages for lay people and identify effective media channels or publishers with a commitment to reaching certain groups of people.

NATIONAL HEALTH-RESEARCH MANAGERS

Successful linkages of research to policy are not a matter of merely changing the attitudes or modifying the skill sets of the researchers themselves. Other mediators are needed. Distinctive contributions may come from people responsible for providing leadership in health research, such as directors of research institutions (including academic institutions), coordinators of national research networks and forums, and executives of funding agencies. Such research managers may come from various backgrounds: research per se, academic life, public-service and private-sector management, or leadership of NGOs.

Given the movement toward a "knowledge economy," it is particularly important for research managers to understand how the production and use of knowledge can contribute to economic and social development. For example, people increasingly recognize that an understanding of local conditions is critical to making programs successful. Combining local and global knowledge is an important mediation skill. Local knowledge includes an understanding of epidemiological trends, cultural patterns, and social structures (for example, who the opinion leaders are in a given community). One must adapt knowledge of "evidence-based interventions" imported from the world's scientific databases to effectively apply them to local realities. Knowledge management for change also includes identifying crucial information needs for national health development and translating these needs into research opportunities to enhance local knowledge and facilitate research to develop new technologies. The latter may involve talking to private investors so that certain technology prototypes get into the manufacturing process.

Countries need to make a systematic effort to develop the leadership skills of their national health-research managers. The ENHR mechanism can play a crucial role in producing research managers who understand the process of innovation dissemination and system change. Such research managers would ensure not only that studies generate good-quality research products but also that these studies examine questions relevant to national health priorities and take into account the perceptions and concerns of the various stakeholders. Moreover, these research managers would look for opportunities and possible entry points or linkages to the decision-making process and keep information flowing between the two processes. They would help researchers obtain the viewpoints of various groups for data analysis and for relevant, useful recommendations. They would also play a crucial role in marketing the research products and working to mobilize other groups to assist the process.

The ENHR mechanism can work with research-funding agencies to increase their awareness of the need for such managers, arguing on the basis of the value added in terms of the research funds already provided. This may convince funding agencies to organize training sessions to increase the number of such research managers. The research manager can be a member of the research team or someone the funding agency selects. Whatever the arrangement, it would clearly require additional resources to enable managers to properly carry out their roles. (Some further suggestions for strengthening the leadership skills of national health-research managers can be found in Chapter 6.)

THE ROLE OF NATIONAL GOVERNMENTS AND THE PRIVATE SECTOR

National governments and the private sector can also play an important role in creating and sustaining effective linkages between research and policy. Cooperative or independent efforts can be useful in improving, for example, infrastructure for social communication. This includes both hardware and human resources. Conventionally, the emphasis has been on hardware, such as telephones, newspapers, television, radio, Internet connections, and computers. Yet, groups of people with common goals and objectives can work together in a type of coalition that helps foster communication in the broader population. Both types of infrastructure require investment and active efforts to create and sustain them.

The information industry (commonly referred to as the media) is an example of a private-sector stakeholder with an important role in linking research and action. By informing the public of research gaps, the media can help to create a demand for research. It can also play a critical role in communicating useful information about new knowledge to the public. In turn, the public can influence political leaders in their support for certain health issues, including research on priority problems.

Of greatest importance are an open society that allows debate on social issues and a government that allocates some financial resources to building proper infrastructure for better social communication. In many countries, however, although investment for physical infrastructure is available, the political culture would have to change to allow open social communication. Some countries have a supportive political culture but limited resources for physical infrastructure. In the latter case, funding agencies may be more readily able to step in to provide financial support for the needed infrastructure and improve the communication of research results to users. It is important, however, to invest in the wider infrastructure, rather than simply targeting a portion of investment to the research community; in other words, it is not enough to provide better access to communication for researchers while the rest of the country still has problems with communication infrastructure.

THE ROLE OF THE INTERNATIONAL RESEARCH COMMUNITY

The international research community can also provide crucial support, both directly and indirectly, for effectively linking research to policy. Connecting researchers from countries with comparable health concerns or those with experience in dealing with similar issues is one form of support. This can result in both information exchange and new contacts with decision-makers. The recently launched Alliance for Health Policy and Systems Research may be able to serve in this role.

Another type of support involves creating opportunities for a broader network of researchers to share experiences and learn from one another. An example of this is the annual Global Forum for Health Research. An example at the regional level is the Tropical Medicine and Public Health Center of the Southeast Asian Ministers of Education Organization. Organizations such as these create a sense of belonging to a larger international research community, and they increase the prestige of research for action in countries where people perceive it as less academic and less valuable to the global knowledge base. However, such an increase in prestige is unlikely to occur without a shift in thinking in the international research community, which needs to better appreciate and contribute to local research.

International agencies supporting health research can reshape their supportive roles to better link research to policy. First, they should put greater effort into reconciling their research agendas with national priorities. This requires an ability to listen to various stakeholder groups and understand their positions, rather than using the agency's considerable financial resources to push its agenda.

A fresh approach is needed to support health research for action. Instead of funding research projects or programs, international donor agencies might fund a national mechanism to promote research to meet national priorities and effectively link the results of research to decision-making and action. Both the mechanism and the research projects would require funds. Furthermore, nationals should be in charge of decision-making concerning the use of research funds. For example, in Tanzania the Swiss government provided an endowment of 200 000 USD to establish a Health Research Users' Trust (NIMR 1999). A consortium of national groups manages this fund. It facilitates communication, disseminates information, and implements research projects in line with Tanzania's recently revised health-research priorities. International funding agencies can further support the learning process of national research mechanisms by facilitating their contacts with other mechanisms sharing similar concerns and goals.

Another approach would be to fund only the operating costs of the national mechanisms themselves, which would then mobilize further technical, financial, and political support for research projects. Neither approach has wide acceptance, however, owing to the concern that once such external funding sources start to support developing countries they will always be required. When donors support a management mechanism, they also tend to raise a concern about national responsibility, but they rarely raise the issue in regard to research projects.

As long as countries do not see the need for health research or do not have the capacity to support it from national budgets, they will require funding from external sources. A failure to convince nationals of the worth of investments in health research is often the reason for a country's dependence on external funding. Donors, however, also need to understand that they can achieve a better research linkage to action through better research management, not merely through making research grants available to do research. Investment in a research management mechanism is a cost-effective approach to helping countries create and make use of research for action.

A somewhat sensitive point needs to be made in regard to the mediating role of the international research community, particularly donor agencies. They commonly demand that a country use international consultants or experts as a condition for loans and grants when they involve large amounts of research funding or are intended to support policy changes. The practice is based mainly on the assumption that having external consultants guide country research will benefit developing countries more and ensure better-quality and more timely results. Certainly this practice is neither illogical nor without its benefits, as pointed out in previous analyses of this issue (Berg 1993). However, international agencies should do this with great caution and weigh the benefits of using external consultants from various angles. Such requirements or conditions on loans can lead countries to reject the work of their own nationals. When faced with a trade-off between a level of quality in research and increased involvement of national researchers, it may be preferable if an international agency chooses the latter, provided that national researchers produce adequate research. Such trade-offs are fewer than people imagine. The final decision will depend on a mix between any existing sense of resentment, the ability of the external experts, the dynamics of the research process, and the nature of the research issues. Although there is no ready-made solution, the crucial message is that international funding agencies need to reexamine their policies and practices related to the use of external experts in country-based research for action.

International donors also need to rethink how they view national researchers. In many cases, they treat national researchers as informants and liaison persons, rather than as researchers with a status equal to that of external consultants. Although such roles are important to the research-for-action process, they do not make full use of the capabilities of national researchers, who often have too little involvement in planning for research. If we believe that the effective linkage of research to action depends on the interaction of the various stakeholders and their involvement, then the ways national researchers enter into each study will impact on the final outcome. In most cases, external experts have only an inadequate understanding of the national context, by far the most crucial component determining both the research process and its outcome. Studies aimed at involving stakeholders, linking research to decision processes, and marketing research products would benefit most from the involvement of national researchers who have a thorough understanding of the local context and the orientations of the various stakeholders. Although not all national researchers can claim to possess such ability and insight, there will always be those who can.

A chapter of the *World Development Report 1998/99: Knowledge for Development* (World Bank 1999) examines the role of international institutions in the production and use of knowledge, including those functioning as "intermediaries":

> *Most knowledge that is beneficial for developing countries is not the product of internationally sponsored research, vital though such research can be. It is rather the consequence of actions taken in developing countries themselves. Local knowledge creation — and its transfer from one country to another — thus has the potential to unleash powerful development forces. Learning from others, assimilating that knowledge, and adapting it to local circumstances offer the opportunity to make rapid advances without repeating others' mistakes.*
>
> — World Bank (1999, p. 133)

In several examples, international health-research agencies have played an important intermediary role in sharing knowledge and experience. COHRED's monograph series is an example of such a contribution, one of compiling and analyzing the experience of developing countries on specific activities (see Chapter 8, Box 8.4). As well, the Kaiser Family Foundation and other agencies provide support to HST in South Africa. Among its publications is the annual *South Africa Health Review*, which provides a record of the struggles, achievements, and challenges of one country as it has tried to implement policies to provide effective and equitable health care to its citizens (HST 1999). Another example is the 1998 Population Reference Bureau review, describing how operations research has contributed to improved reproductive-health services in various parts of the world (see Box 5.6). The recently created cluster on Evidence and Information for Policy at the World Health Organization provides

> **Box 5.6**
>
> ### How can operations research improve reproductive health?
>
> Operations research focuses on policies and the day-to-day operations of programs. It includes pilot projects to try out new strategies and approaches to service delivery, evaluations of existing programs to pinpoint problems and recommend solutions, and experiments to test the impacts and cost-effectiveness of various solutions. The active participation of program managers and policymakers in operations research, from the identification of a problem through to its resolution, helps to ensure the usefulness of research.
>
> A 1998 publication by the Population Reference Bureau described a number of ways in which operations research has improved reproductive health:
>
> **Improving quality of care**
> Operations research helps to determine what aspects of quality are most important to clients and providers. It has, for example, given program managers information about the dynamics of family-planning-method use, including how to reduce discontinuation rates, effectively introduce new methods, expand the method mix, and better understand method switching.
>
> **Reaching special populations**
> Operations research can help program managers and policymakers identify special groups that, for a variety of reasons, have not been served by traditional family-planning programs and test innovative strategies to reach them.
>
> **Integrating reproductive-health services**
> Programs that provide a range of integrated reproductive-health services have gained popularity among managers and planners of family-planning programs. It is thought that integrated services may be more cost-effective than separate services, and they may better meet the needs of clients and lead to better overall client health. Operations research is helping to test these assumptions and guide the combination and delivery of integrated services.
>
> **Increasing sustainability**
> Making programs sustainable without substantial external assistance has become a priority in many countries. Operations research has helped to determine the relative cost-effectiveness of alternative approaches and test ways to streamline program activities while maintaining quality services.
>
> Source: Chalkley and Shane (1998).

useful information to guide policy development at both global and national levels. Most of the work to date has concentrated on producing interesting information on developing countries' health situations, but with relatively little involvement of national researchers.

CONCLUSION

In many countries, the focus of research for action has been on strengthening researchers' communication skills, but such initiatives rely on the overly simplistic assumption that proper packaging ensures the best use of research. To increase the likelihood of research leading to action, we need to include many other factors in the equation. One is that the research-planning process requires broader participation and a diversity of dynamics. Another is that researchers need to concern themselves with the decision-making process and become involved in it, rather than paying attention solely to their research. They also need to improve their communication of research results, adopting more of a social-marketing approach.

To enable such a holistic participatory approach to yield the best results, researchers and research users need to strengthen their capabilities. A national mechanism with a dynamic, interactive, and inclusive process would be crucial to improving the chances of research linking successfully to action. The research community, decision-makers, and research-funding agencies need leaders, or managers, who understand the concepts and practices of knowledge management for change. Government also has a critical role to play, especially in providing both physical and social infrastructure to facilitate or demand research for action. The international research community and funding agencies need to change many of their conventional attitudes and practices and look at research for action more from a country viewpoint and from that of longer term development goals.

CHAPTER 6

FOSTERING A NATIONAL CAPACITY FOR EQUITY-ORIENTED HEALTH RESEARCH

Victor Neufeld

SUMMARY

In its report, the Commission on Health Research for Development emphasized the importance of capacity-building for country-specific health research. What have been the achievements over the past 10 years in building national capacity to both produce and use equity-oriented health research, particularly in low-income countries? This is the central question addressed in this chapter. Following an analysis of this question, it goes on to present some lessons from the initiatives of the past decade and to propose strategies to guide future action.

WHAT HAS BEEN ACHIEVED?

To indicate trends and draw conclusions from a range of diverse efforts, several case studies are presented in this chapter. At the global level, it examines the capacity-strengthening activities of two programs: the Special Programme for Research and Training in Tropical Diseases (TDR) and the International Clinical Epidemiology Network (INCLEN). It examines regional initiatives, including the training activities of the Tropical Medicine and Public Health Center network of the Southeast Asian Ministers of Education Organization (SEAMEO–TROPMED) and an initiative to analyze malaria-research capacity in Africa, conducted as a contribution to the Multilateral Initiative on Malaria (MIM). At the national level, it describes a 1998 study of capacity development for health research in Uganda and complements this with six brief country profiles of health-research capacity-strengthening activities.

Several types of evidence are considered to determine whether efforts over the past decade have indeed strengthened national health-research systems. Although it is difficult to make a direct causal link, it would appear that the global burden of illness borne by the poor has not decreased substantially in the past decade and that the global investment in health research (including capacity-strengthening) directed to the problems of the poor and disadvantaged has not increased substantially over the same 10 years. The available data suggest a mixed picture of research-related human-resource development and its deployment to meet the needs of low-income countries. Although the return rate of scientists to their own countries from the major training programs looks encouraging, the brain drain continues (both to developed countries and to transnational corporations within developing countries). Furthermore, the quality of the research environment is still a major impediment to enhancing and sustaining efforts in most low-income countries.

This chapter also briefly examines several output indicators. Although the percentage of scientific contributions from low-income countries to the global health knowledge base has increased slightly, the predominant pattern of the past 10 years continues to be one of imbalance. An overwhelming proportion of global scientific output is contributed by scientists in industrialized countries and focuses on the health problems of the North.

Wide disparities remain, therefore, between the research capacity of low-income countries and that of middle- to high-income ones. Also apparent is the need for more relevant and comprehensive information to evaluate activities in research capacity-strengthening. One encouraging sign is a renewed interest in the issue of health inequity and the need to accelerate research, and its application, on this fundamental issue. Also, awareness is growing among international agencies of the need to strengthen research capacities at the national level.

WHAT HAS BEEN LEARNED?

Five lessons can be learned from the capacity-strengthening experience of the past 10 years:

— Capacity-development activities should be more country driven;

— The focus has been too narrow, restricted mostly to individuals and institutions (the need is for a broader national-systems approach);

- The predominant emphasis has been on a supply-side approach, with relatively little attention to demand-driven capacity development;
- Capacity-strengthening programs and policies should pay more attention to the goal of equity in health; and
- Capacity-strengthening initiatives should put more emphasis on fostering broad problem-solving competencies across the whole spectrum of the research process.

WHAT CAN BE DONE BETTER IN THE FUTURE?

The goal for the next decade remains unchanged: it is to ensure that all societies, particularly those in low-income countries, have the capacity to apply both local and global knowledge to their own health and development problems, particularly those of poor and disadvantaged people. As a corollary, it follows that these same countries, given the opportunity, would have much to contribute to the global understanding of health and development. The following are four elements of a more efficient framework for achieving this goal:

- New research and learning coalitions at both national and subnational levels to address high-priority health and development problems;
- New tools to set health-research priorities, assess health equity, monitor resource flows, and evaluate efforts to develop capacity;
- New leadership, both individual and collective, with a focus on special competencies such as creating demand, building coalitions, developing leadership per se, and managing knowledge, with the latter including the ability to harness the potential benefits of the new information and communication technologies (ICTs); and
- New forms of partnership, which are sorely needed, particularly between countries and institutions of the North and South (these must be truly collaborative relationships, based on mutual respect and shared goals).

INTRODUCTION

"Strengthening research capacity in developing countries is one of the most powerful, cost effective and sustainable means of advancing health and development" (CHRD 1990, p. 71). This is the bold and sweeping first sentence of the chapter "Building and Sustaining Research Capacity" in the Commission's 1990 report. It reflects the optimistic premise that has characterized health-research capacity-building efforts since the 1970s. At that time, encouraged by the gains made through research against smallpox, polio, and other diseases, the global scientific community confidently believed that more research would soon lead us to understand and eradicate other microbial diseases — perhaps most of them. Poor countries, situated for the most part in tropical climates, would be the most important beneficiaries. And so thousands of scientists from low-income countries received specialized training to do research on the "major killers," such as malaria and other endemic infectious diseases.

By 1990, the Commission concluded that despite two decades of effort,

> *far too little attention is being given to the critical importance of building and sustaining individuals and institutional health research capacity within developing countries. To remedy this problem, leadership and commitment by national governments as well as longer-term support by international agencies will be necessary.*
>
> CHRD (1990, p. 85)

The specific conclusions on capacity-building from chapter 8 of the Commission's report are presented in Box 6.1. In the final chapter of the Commission's report it urged, as part of the recommendations on Essential National Health Research (ENHR), that every country develop a national health-research plan. The recommendation included the following statement:

> *Implementing such a plan will require building and maintaining research capacity within developing countries and sustained reinforcement from the international community. A critical mass of health researchers is needed in every country, nurtured by improved career paths, including incentives and rewards. The research capacity should be closely linked to the policymakers, managers and other users of the results of research. Government support is essential.*
>
> CHRD (1990, pp. 85–86)

In the same year, the theme of the World Health Assembly (WHA) was the role of health research in the strategy to promote Health for All by the Year 2000. The resolutions of this 43rd WHA (Davies and

> **Box 6.1**
>
> **Commission conclusions on building and sustaining research capacity**
>
> 1. Building and sustaining research capacity within developing countries is an essential and effective means of accelerating research contributions to health and development. Nurturing individual scientific competence and leadership, strengthening institutions, establishing strong linkages between research and action agencies, and reinforcing national institutions through international networks are all important elements of capacity building.
> 2. Capacity building for country-specific health research should be given top priority by every country because of its importance to policy and management decisions for the health sector. It is equally important to create demand for research results among those responsible for health policy and management through effective arrangements for communication and shared priority setting for research.
> 3. National commitment is indispensable to secure the resources and to create a positive environment for research capacity building.
> 4. Bilateral and multilateral agencies and development banks should reduce their dependence on expatriate consultants and increase their investment in research capacity in developing countries. Special attention should be given to sub-Saharan African countries.
> 5. Capacity building requires sustained support over an extended period. External agencies can assist more effectively by committing at the outset support for 10 to 15 years subject only to demonstrating achievement in relation to agreed-upon milestones and normal agency legal and reporting requirements.
>
> Source: CHRD (1990, p. 79).

Mansourian 1992) included several specific recommendations about research capacity-strengthening:

- URGES *member states, particularly developing countries: ... to build and strengthen national research capabilities by investing resources in national institutions, by providing appropriate career opportunities to attract and retain the involvement of their own scientists, and by creating environments that will foster scholarship and creativity;*

- URGES *bilateral and multilateral development agencies, non-governmental organizations, foundations and appropriate regional organizations: ... to increase their support for essential health research, and research capability building.*

Now, 10 years later, what can the global health-research community say about another decade of activity? More specifically, what have been the achievements in building national capacity to produce and use equity-oriented health research, particularly in low-income countries?

Paying special attention to these features, this chapter devotes a section to each of the following questions:

— What has been achieved in the past 10 years?

— What are the key lessons from the initiatives of the past decade?

— What strategies can be considered to guide future efforts?

WHAT HAS BEEN ACHIEVED?

To begin the exploration of this question, it may be useful to look at examples (case studies) of efforts to develop health-research capacity over the past decade. It is not the intention here to present a comprehensive in-depth analysis. Rather, by examining several diverse efforts, we can observe trends and draw some conclusions. Also, the reality is that efforts to develop health-research capacity in the past decade have been diverse. Although diversity has its benefits, the aggregate global capacity-development effort is still fragmented. This can be seen in the sources of any given initiative (for example, country or external agency), the lack of coordination among external agencies and networks, and the variable focus (for example, institution, discipline, disease). The examples selected for this chapter include two global programs — one supported by multilateral agencies — and one supported by a foundation; two regional initiatives; and a national study and some country "snapshots" of research capacity-strengthening.

RESEARCH CAPACITY-STRENGTHENING ACTIVITIES OF TDR

Cosponsored by the United Nations Development Programme (UNDP), the World Bank, and the World Health Organization (WHO) and supported by other agencies, TDR began operations in 1976. In most of these operations, it has addressed eight tropical diseases through research and development (R&D) directly and through capacity-strengthening (it should be noted that it recently added tuberculosis and dengue to its list). In the Commission's 1990 report, it recommended "continuing and expanded support" (CHRD 1990, p. 88) for the TDR program, along with another WHO-associated initiative, the Special Programme of Research, Development and Research Training in Human Reproduction (HRP). The main elements of TDR's research capacity-strengthening component include grants for research training (more than 1 300 since 1976), for reentry (about 300 during this same period), and for institution-strengthening (266 during this time). The total financial investment has been more than 100 million USD.

Major reviews of research capacity-strengthening activities were conducted in 1990 (WHO 1991) and again in 1998 (as part of an external review of TDR) (TDR 1998). The 1992 review, done in collaboration with HRP and the Global Programme on AIDS, paid special attention to least-developed countries (LDCs) — the 42 countries where the per capita gross national product is less than 300 USD/year. Although TDR had supported research capacity-strengthening activities in nine of these countries, the general consensus was that the overall contribution of the three participating WHO programs to the research capacity of LDCs left much to be desired. This report recommended a 12-month initial action plan, in which three to six countries would have special attention, with the stated expectation that the three WHO-associated programs and the interim Task Force on Health Research for Development (charged with facilitating ENHR) would collaborate actively.

The more recent review recognized that the available evidence concerned process and outcome indicators, which led to the following conclusion: "One could observe that the RCS [research capacity-strengthening] programme operates well, that its trainees graduate, that investigators publish, and that technology is transferred. The question of impact requires further thought" (Wayling 1999, p. 6). The 1998 report of the External Review Committee made no reference to the 1992 expectations of collaborative focus on three to six LDCs but made the following statement: "The Committee felt that there was now an increasing urgency to develop more effective strategies to meet the capacity development needs of the least developed countries and to focus on developing countries bearing the largest burden of disease" (TDR 1998, p. 45).

TDR is a good example of sustained collaborative support from three agencies focused on specific disease conditions. The capacity-building strategy has concentrated primarily on individuals and institutions in disease-specific research. Until the 1992 review, strengthening national health-research systems enjoyed little emphasis, particularly in low-income countries. The 1998 third external review included the following as one of two "mandatory" recommendations: "more focused strategies are needed to strengthen the research capacity of countries and regions bearing the heaviest burden of endemic tropical diseases, with an increasing focus on least developed countries" (TDR 1998, p. 6). By 2000, overall funding for research capacity-strengthening in LDCs was 33%. Evaluative efforts to date have featured process and outcome indicators. The available reports have not included evidence on whether the global burden of disease for the conditions in the TDR portfolio has diminished incrementally since the program began 25 years ago.

THE INTERNATIONAL CLINICAL EPIDEMIOLOGY NETWORK

In the late 1970s, Kerr White, an outspoken supporter of clinical epidemiology, became increasingly concerned about the continuing schism between clinical medicine and public health (White 1991). At the same time, the Rockefeller Foundation was reviewing its investment in health-science institutions, and its report concluded that "the most pressing problem in the broader field of health ... is more effective management of health services at all levels" (Evans 1981, p. 11). In addition, this report concluded that "those who might provide leadership and management lack the inclination, breadth of perspective, and analytic skills to respond to this challenge" (Evans 1981, p. 11). In 1982, these concerns led to the creation of INCLEN, which the Rockefeller Foundation initiated and supports. A progress report for INCLEN appeared in 1991 (Halstead et al. 1991).

The key strategy of INCLEN has been to carefully select young professionals from designated academic institutions in developing countries, provide them with training in clinical-epidemiological research, and support the creation of clinical-epidemiological units (CEUs) within universities. A critical mass of INCLEN trainees (usually about 6–10) staff the CEUs. Most of the trainees are clinicians, and the hope is that these young medical practitioners will contribute to solving health-care problems in their respective countries. Over time, INCLEN added special training elements in health economics and health social sciences (Higginbotham 1992). Recognizing that the Rockefeller Foundation would eventually withdraw its financial support, INCLEN began to operate as an independent nonprofit organization in 1991.

Over the almost two decades since INCLEN began, it has given training in research methods in clinical epidemiology and related fields to about 500 professionals. Fifty-four institutions from 28 countries have been involved. INCLEN has received more than 75 million

USD from the Rockefeller Foundation and some additional funds from other sources (about 10 million USD).

A 1999 external-review team recognized INCLEN's strong contributions to education and research in clinical epidemiology. In addition to making several strategic recommendations regarding INCLEN's future, the review recommended a stronger engagement in the broader field of public health and urged the organization to consider Africa a planning-priority region. INCLEN is currently undergoing a major transition, strengthening regional networks and shifting its leadership to health professionals "living in countries with the greatest burden of disease" (Macfarlane et al. 2000, p. 503).

INCLEN has provided strong technical training in health-research methods. A number of former INCLEN faculty now hold senior positions in universities, ministries of health, and international organizations. Several INCLEN faculty have contributed strongly to the promotion, advocacy, and implementation of ENHR. Like TDR, INCLEN has a strategic focus on training individuals and creating and supporting institutional units (the CEUs). It has produced a cadre of indigenous researchers capable of carrying out their own research, and in this way it has strengthened the national human-resource base for health research. It has also developed strong regional networks (in clinical epidemiology). However, the issue of national health-research capacity-strengthening has not been an explicit priority in INCLEN's training and research activities. One might also note that it has invested in only 2 of the 42 WHO-designated LDCs — Ethiopia and Uganda.

REGIONAL INITIATIVES

SEAMEO–TROPMED network

More than 30 years ago, the governments of Southeast Asia established SEAMEO–TROPMED and aimed it at reducing the burden of illness in the subregion (more information is available from http://www.tm.mahidol.ac.th/menu.htm). One of the network's objectives is "to support research on endemic and newly emerging diseases that are associated with changing environment and lifestyle" (CHRD 1990, p. 78). It has designated four institutions as TROPMED Regional Centres; they are located in host institutions in Jakarta, Kuala Lumpur, Manila, and Bangkok. Over these 30 years, more than 3 500 medical and allied health professionals have received training in various subspecialties of tropical medicine and public health. Cooperation arrangements with institutions in industrialized countries have provided supplementary expertise, as needed. The network serves as a link to bilateral and multilateral assistance programs under WHO and other United Nations agencies.

TROPMED's research-capacity program has had no formal assessment. However, information is available about the number of proposals funded and completed, publication patterns, and research-funding trends. The report of WHO's April 2000 meeting on research capacity-strengthening, held in Annecy, France, stated that "TROPMED alumni have distinguished themselves in both the public and private service sectors — as administrators, outstanding scientists, academicians, health practitioners, technocrats, and national leaders" (WHO 2000c, p. 5). Since 1990 most of TROPMED's training efforts have focused on the basic knowledge and skills for research design and methodology to support the specific national health programs of SEAMEO member countries; exceptions are Indonesia, Malaysia, Philippines, and Thailand, which are already quite advanced in this regard. This network is a good example of the value of cooperation among countries in the same region. In fact, the eight ministers of education who originally founded the network believed that cooperation among Asian countries (in this case, focused on tropical medicine and public health) is vital to the region's prosperity and stability.

Malaria research in Africa

MIM is a global initiative concerned particularly with building malaria-research capacity in Africa to address the increasing threat of this disease. As part of the initiative, Wellcome Trust recently published a study to assess Africa's capacity for malaria research (Beattie et al. 1999). The study surveyed training opportunities and provided an assessment of capacity and training. Some of the key findings were as follows:

- Using the Science Citation Index (SCI) database, an analysis of malaria publications for the period of 1995–97 revealed that 17.2% of the articles had an African address. The United States contributed 30% of all malaria publications globally; the United Kingdom, 17.8%; and France, 9.6%. During this same period, the contribution of Africa to overall research in health and biomedicine was only 1.2% of the world's output. Of additional interest is that the 1 000 articles on malaria published in 1995 represented only 0.3% of all articles in the SCI, compared with 10.2% for cardiology and 2.4% for arthritis and rheumatism.

- Of the 752 malaria researchers working in 52 centres in Africa at the time of the study, 192 (26%) were postdoctoral scientists, and 168 (22%) were clinicians. They were dispersed across 22 countries. About one-third of Africa's malaria research groups were led by nonnational scientists.

- The study attempted to measure the impact of research through an analysis of the malaria management guidelines and policies of 11 African countries. This proved difficult because much of the evidence used for policy was in "grey literature." Also, many of the bibliographies in policy documents were incomplete.

- For the 5-year period of 1993–98, the study found that 88% of malaria-research grants awarded to Africa researchers came from organizations outside the continent. For PhD training, 65% of acknowledgments were to industrialized-country agencies, and 17% were to African governments or local sources.

The report gave several recommendations of particular relevance to the issue of fostering national capacity; it made a strong plea for "overarching mechanisms" to match capacity development to national research priorities and recommended that initiatives continue to prepare African scientific leaders to hold major roles in the future.

COUNTRY INITIATIVES

A country case study: capacity development for health research in Uganda

In 1998, the Board of the Council on Health Research for Development (COHRED) decided to review its strategy for ENHR capacity development. Part of this review involved country consultations and studies; Uganda did one of these studies (UCD 1998). This was a timely initiative for Uganda, as the country had considerable experience with implementing the ENHR approach, including applying this approach at the district level. In addition, it had recently developed a new ENHR plan (with a revision of health-research priorities); however, the capacity-development component of the plan was weak and required strengthening and specification.

The study had three objectives:

— To review Uganda's current capacity to conduct, use, and manage priority-driven health research;

— To use the results of this review to develop a capacity-development plan as an integral component of Uganda's new ENHR plan; and

— To contribute to an international exploration of capacity development for ENHR.

The study team used several methods to conduct this review, including a standardized interview-based survey of health organizations and institutions, with both producers and users of research; a Medline search of Ugandan health-research publications; and an analysis of health-research projects registered in the database of the Uganda National Council for Science and Technology.

A striking observation was that virtually all of the funding for research (more than 99%) came from external sources. Although much of the research in Uganda was on the recently revised health-research priority themes, many researchers were unaware of these priorities; it also appeared that donors were equally unaware of them. Most health-research organizations in Uganda shared the goal of conducting and using research to improve the health of Uganda's citizens. Although the actual number of researchers was considerable, a number of major barriers stood in the way of Uganda's effective deployment of this "pool" of competent individuals, such as competing demands, weak infrastructure, limited and irregular funding, and low professional recognition. Although many research projects were at the district level, the study team felt that COHRED could do much more to involve district-level groups and organizations at all stages of the research. The team fully recognized the need to create a national health-research network (or organization) to facilitate interactions among stakeholders and provide overall coordination.

The study team presented these findings at a national workshop, which put forward several specific recommendations. In particular, it strongly supported the creation of the Uganda National Health Research Organization (UNHRO). Some personnel shifts at the Ministry of Health, made shortly after the workshop, delayed action on most of the recommendations. Although the UNHRO initiative is now back on track, the government has still not ratified the organization as an official parastatal body. In part, this is because the Government of Uganda is busy with the next phase of its evolving political system. UNHRO is nevertheless functioning on an interim basis, with some support from the Ugandan government, and has responsibility for several specific tasks, such as strengthening a national health-research database, organizing an annual health-research forum, facilitating district-level research (beginning with several "demonstration districts"), and refining a health-research plan within the current national health plan.

The Ugandan story illustrates the vulnerability of good plans (prepared by good people) to local political shifts. However, it is also a tribute to a small cadre of individuals who, despite considerable odds, have persisted in nurturing the vision of a national health-research system responsive to the needs of the Ugandan people.

"Snapshots" from other countries

Several other low- to middle-income countries have conducted reviews of their national health-research capacities. Some of these reviews were presented and discussed at the Annecy meeting. Others were national initiatives of other kinds. Summarized below are some of the highlights of these reviews.

— *Pakistan* — Created in 1962, the Pakistan Medical Research Council has been more active in the last several years on national health research: it has conducted workshops on research methodology, organized a biennial research congress, and sponsored several national conferences on specific issues. An example of these efforts is a conference to discuss the findings and policy implications of a national health-research survey. The report (presented at the Annecy meeting) stated that Pakistan had made "no discernible progress with the development of health research capacity" (Akhtar 2000, p. 1). It also described the "health bureaucracy" as lacking interest in health research and as being sceptical of its importance. This reflects an overall lack of "research culture" in the country, and the report recognized the need for long-term planning, including an overhaul of the educational system itself, to bring about a change in thinking and behaviour.

— *Kenya* — In 1998, Kenya conducted a major review of its national health-research activities of the previous 5 years, including an analysis of activities in research capacity-strengthening. The review recognized that Kenya had many highly qualified researchers, working in several research institutions and organizations, but concluded that capacity-development activities needed to include a broader range of stakeholders. It made specific recommendations for developing community leaders and strengthening links with the private sector. In addition, it noted that Kenya had recently put more emphasis on helping researchers develop competencies and skills in all aspects of the research process, with a view to complementing "core" expertise in particular disciplines.

— *Indonesia* — An analysis of health-research capacity-strengthening was a component of Indonesia's recently revised National Policy on Health Research and Development. Led by its National Institute of Health Research and Development, Indonesia has prepared a national health-research agenda, strengthened its health-research network, and provided opportunities for guided research training at various levels. It has recognized that decision-makers and health-research managers should make a more explicit commitment to capacity-strengthening and that donor agencies need a forum to create specific collaborative arrangements for realistically responding to the capacity-development needs of the national health-research system.

— *Lao PDR* — In 1992, after recovering from a costly and devastating war, the Government of Lao PDR turned its attention to creating a master health plan. Health research was one of nine components of this 5-year plan. To develop human resources for research was a major goal during this period. The activities for this purpose included holding various training workshops, creating collaborative research arrangements with other countries in the region, encouraging publication of reports and articles, and introducing research training into the university curriculum. Health research again features prominently in the current health plan, which includes responses to lessons learned from the previous 5 years, such as the importance of integrating health research into health-system management at all levels, strengthening the incentive system for researchers, and involving policy- and decision-makers in research activities. The report (presented at the Annecy meeting) also included a list of further challenges. It recognized that research is vital to realizing expected health gains and, in particular, vital to assuring "equity in health and

- *Tanzania* — Over the past 2 years, Tanzania has taken some important steps to strengthen its national health-research system. It created a multistakeholder National Health Research Forum in 1998. In 1999, it undertook a major effort to revise national health-research priorities. These developments took place in the context of a comprehensive program of national health-sector reform. Tanzania has recognized it has a capacity gap in health-research management and leadership. A national workshop in January 2000 gave a venue for discussion of this gap, which led Tanzania to initiate a planning process for capacity development in health research. The country is conducting capacity inventories at various levels and has a major initiative under way to establish a research-support system for district-based health and development.

- *Myanmar* — Through the Department of Medical Research in the Ministry of Health, Myanmar has made considerable progress over the past 10 years in strengthening its health-research capacity. Official policy statements have recognized the importance of research. A variety of training opportunities are available to individuals. The country has conducted various institutional-development activities, such as national seminars on research management and the enhancement of the use of research findings. It has identified several needs. For example, the report (also presented at the Annecy meeting) stated that "the most serious factor hindering research in Myanmar is the need to further enhance a research culture, ... [including] an abiding belief in research as a necessary tool for development" (Pang Soe and Than Tuu 2000, p. 11).

These case studies and country stories are illustrative of various aspects of health-research capacity-strengthening over the past 10 years, including a long-standing program sponsored by multilateral agencies, a global network funded largely by a single foundation, two regional initiatives, a national initiative in Uganda, and the national initiatives of several other countries.

ANALYSIS OF THE EVIDENCE

What is the evidence that the efforts of the past decade have actually strengthened national health-research systems in low-income countries for the purpose of benefiting poor and disadvantaged people? The remainder of this section considers four types of evidence (among various possible data sources) on this question.

Burden of disease

Have investments in health in the past 10 years lessened the burden of disease among the poor in low-income countries? Obviously, given the growing realization that many factors, in addition to the interventions of the health system itself, determine ill-health, it is impossible or inappropriate to directly link changes in the burden of disease with levels of investment in health research. However, it is possible to put two general statements side by side and consider some implications:

— The global burden of disease borne by the poor has not decreased substantially during the decade of the 1990s; and

— The global investment in health research directed to the problems of the poor and disadvantaged has not increased substantially over the same decade.

It should be emphasized that these statements are very preliminary and intentionally provocative. One can expect the participants at the October 2000 conference to debate more detailed information on each of these statements.

In recent work on the global burden of disease among the poor, Gwatkin and others (Gwatkin et al. 1999; Gwatkin and Guillot 2000) reanalyzed the Murray–Lopez reports on the global disease burden. Using various types of distributional analyses (that is, comparing the richest and poorest groups), they found that the poor are still burdened mostly with communicable diseases. They extrapolated that a faster decline in communicable diseases would decrease the poor–rich gap, whereas a faster decline in noncommunicable illnesses would increase this gap. If health inequity is the pervading concern, investments in health research (including capacity-strengthening) and action should, for the foreseeable future, remain priorities on the "unfinished agenda" on communicable diseases.

Recently, WHO prepared a brief entitled "Health: a Precious Asset" (WHO 2000a), as a contribution to the June 2000 special session of the United Nations General Assembly (called Copenhagen

Plus Five). At this meeting, the United Nations reviewed progress on commitments made at the 1995 World Summit for Social Development. The report of this meeting included the following sobering admission: "we must frankly acknowledge that the poor quality or, in some instances the absence, of data is a significant obstacle to tracking the health status of the poor (WHO 2000a, p. 9). It went on to present some of the available evidence concerning "the health revolution that left out a billion people" (WHO 2000a, p. 9) and summarized some tables from *The World Health Report 1999* (WHO 1999) concerning the health status of the poor versus that of the nonpoor, using 1990 data. It then described how certain major health conditions (HIV–AIDS, malaria, tuberculosis, malnutrition, maternal mortality, and others) all hit hardest on the poor and vulnerable. In a section entitled "Health Services in Decline," it described inequities between and within countries. One section of the report began with the assertion that "the delivery of health care itself is often profoundly antipoor" (WHO 1999, p. 13). Within WHO's proposals for action, two of WHO's own contributions would be to

— Build country capacities to assess the impacts of economic, technological, cultural, and political aspects of globalization on health equity and the health status of poor and vulnerable people and design responses to these impacts; and

— Build a global knowledge base on social development in health and on good practices in the protection and improvement of the health status of poor and vulnerable people.

The current global knowledge base cannot tell us clearly whether our collective efforts of the past decade have actually strengthened the health-research systems of low-income countries enough to lessen the burden of disease on poor and vulnerable people.

Human resources

Have the development and deployment of human resources for health research over the past 10 years responded to the needs of low income countries? TDR and INCLEN have presented some encouraging findings on the brain-drain concern. TDR reported that only 4.5% (6/131) of those who earned PhDs between 1990 and 1997 failed to return to their home country after completing training. Over 25 years, the return rate of TDR-sponsored trainees was 97% (Wayling 1999). During the first phase of INCLEN in 1992 (when all training occurred in industrialized-country centres), it estimated that 10% of trainees failed to complete their studies or failed to return to their home sponsoring institutions (Lansang, personal communication, 2000[1]).

However, a recent study conducted by the United Nations Educational, Scientific and Cultural Organization found that many African PhD graduates were living outside of Africa (about 30 000) (UNESCO 1999). A 1992 study counted only 20 000 scientists and engineers in Africa — 0.36% of the world total (UNESCO 1999). The *Human Development Report 1999* has tables displaying the number of R&D scientists and technicians per 1 000 people for 1990–96 (UNDP 1999). This ratio was 1.3 for the world, 4.1 for industrialized countries, and 0.4 for developing countries — no data were available for the LDCs. The *World Development Report 1998/99* gave similar information, showing the number of scientists and engineers in R&D per million people for 1981–95 (World Bank 1999). Again, for many developing countries, the data were unavailable. All the available estimates of this number for some low-income countries set it at less than 100, whereas it is higher than 2 000 for most industrialized countries.

Any discussion in a developing country about human resources for health research touches on the issue of the "internal brain drain." This is the phenomenon of individuals being "pirated" to work within their own countries by multinational pharmaceutical companies and international health agencies. In many developing countries, this phenomenon has resulted in low national health-research capacity and a small number of well-trained and competent individuals being "stretched thin," taking on a variety of responsibilities.

Although some general studies of the "external brain drain" are available (Carrington and Detragiache 1999), comprehensive information at the national level regarding human resources for health research is lacking. In-depth national studies would be very helpful. In particular, one needs information not only on the numbers of researchers but also on the quality of their research time and whether they are allocating that time to addressing priority health concerns in their countries. Countries should integrate this kind of information into the capacity-development component of their health-research plans and programs. Numerous recent discussions with national health-research leaders have indicated that major challenges remain in enhancing and sustaining the research environment in low-income countries.

---

[1] M.A. Lansang, Philippine Society for Microbiology and Infectious Diseases, Quezon City, Philippines, personal communication, 2000.

Outputs

In a 1995 article in the popular magazine *Scientific American*, Gibbs gave an analysis of the contributions of researchers from low-income countries to the world's scientific literature (Gibbs 1995). The key finding was that low-income countries are "nearly invisible" in the world's most influential scientific journals. He went on to suggest that this situation reflects "the economics and biases of science publishing as much as the actual quality of Third World research" (Gibbs 1995, p. 93). At the April 2000 Annecy meeting, Gibbs presented an update on this issue. The number of accessible journals in the new

> *Web of Science/SCI-E is now large — more than 5,500 journals compared to about 3,500 journals in the 1995 Science Citation Index database. This has increased the number of papers authored by scientists from low and middle-income countries — for example, from India, Malaysia and Brazil — identified in such surveys. The number of journals from these countries included in the larger database is also "inching up" slowly. However, access by developing country research institutions to this database is decreasing; several journal donation programs have been discontinued — an example is a long-standing program sponsored by the American Association for the Advancement of Science.*
>
> Gibbs (1995, p. 93)

Will the ICT revolution enable scientists from low-income countries to more equitably access and contribute to the global knowledge base on health? There are promising signs. For example, the *British Medical Journal* has broadened its editorial board to include several members from developing countries. This journal (and an increasing number of others) is now accessible electronically and for free. Several journals based in industrialized countries now actively commission news and articles relevant to the health situation of developing countries.

Another measure of progress in national research capacity-strengthening may be the increase in the numbers of actually funded and completed research projects and, perhaps more importantly, a greater focus in research activity on national health-research priorities. In the Uganda study (described above), the annual number of projects did not change during the 5-year study (1993–97). Almost all the projects in the registry related in one way or another to six predetermined priority areas, with about two-thirds focusing on communicable diseases and the largest percentage of these on AIDS. Analyses in other countries have given similar findings — for example, the Philippines (COHRED 1997c).

What can we learn from this brief look at research outputs (specifically projects and publications)? In general, the scientific outputs of the industrialized countries contribute overwhelmingly to the global knowledge base, as measured in numbers of journal articles. Consistent with the "10/90 disequibilibrium," a phrase usually used to describe financial flows, only a small percentage of the world's scientific literature on health concerns the health problems of 90% of the world's people.

Funding

What progress has been made over the past 10 years on the objective of allocating a more equitable proportion of health-research funding (including funding for capacity-strengthening) to low-income countries and to research on the health conditions of the poor? It may be useful to return to the Commission's report. Using 1986 data, the Commission estimated that only 5% of an estimated 30 billion USD was directed to finding solutions to the main health problems of 95% of the world's population. This situation led the Commission to make specific recommendations on ways to mobilize research funding:

— Developing countries should invest at least 2% of national health expenditures in research and in research capacity-strengthening, and

— Aid agencies should earmark at least 5% of their project and program aid for the health sector for research and research capacity-strengthening.

In addition to making these quantitative recommendations, the Commission also made suggestions about the quality of research and of research capacity-strengthening efforts, such as longer term funding, innovative financing strategies, and broader support.

A review was conducted 5 years later for WHO's Ad Hoc Committee on Health Research Relating to Future Intervention Options, using a 1992 estimate of global funding for health R&D (at 55.8 billion USD). The review found that the problem was getting worse, with only 4.4% (2.4 billion USD) directed to addressing the health problems of low- to middle-income countries (Ad Hoc Committee 1996). An update of the global situation will be presented at the October 2000 Bangkok conference.

At a regional level, the Pan American Health Organization has an ongoing project to help countries monitor resource flows and obtain alternative funding. The project, known as Opportunities for

Health Research Financing, recently analyzed 26 Inter-American Development Bank (IDB) projects between 1992 and 1990 on their health-research component (Panisset 1999). Of all IDB-sector loans, 6.7% went to research (totaling about 260 000 USD). Subanalysis at a country level revealed wide ranges. For example, in Brazil 23% of loan resources went to research; in Argentina, the proportion was only 5%.

Recently, COHRED's Task Force on Resource Flows undertook national studies of resource flows for health R&D in Malaysia, the Philippines, and Thailand (COHRED 2000a). In the Philippines in 1996, 19% of the government budget went to health, but the R&D allocation was less than 1%, and the allocation to health research was 17% of the R&D budget, or 1% of the health budget. Private hospitals and government academic institutions used just more than half of this amount (55%).

What can we conclude from the analysis up to this point? What progress has been made in strengthening the capacity of low-income countries to produce and use research to decrease the burden of disease on poor and disadvantaged people? One obvious conclusion is that developing countries need more and better information. Overall, wide disparities remain between the research capacities of low-income countries and those of middle- to high-income countries.

There are some encouraging signs. Clearly renewed interest and concern are appearing at many levels in the issue of health inequities and the need to do something about them. As described in Chapter 2, the health-research community is actively engaged in analyzing this problem and proposing directions for action. In addition, international organizations are increasingly aware of the need to concentrate capacity-strengthening efforts at a national level. This also appears in the mission and activities of the recently created Alliance for Health Policy and Systems Research (for more information visit http://www.who.int/evidence/alliance.htm), the work of COHRED (1994), and the recent INCLEN transition, which features strengthened regional and national activities.

WHAT HAS BEEN LEARNED?

What has been learned from the capacity-strengthening initiatives of the past 10 years? The following are five suggested lessons:

— Capacity-development activities should be more country driven;

- The focus has been too narrow, restricted mostly to individuals, groups (critical mass), and institutions (a broader systems approach is needed);
- The supply-side model has predominated, leading the capacity-strengthening activities of the past 10 years to neglect the task of creating a capacity to use (and demand) research;
- Capacity-development programs and policies should pay more attention to the goal of equity in health; and
- Capacity-development initiatives should put more emphasis on fostering broad problem-solving competencies in all aspects of research, to complement the more technical elements.

THE IMPORTANCE OF COUNTRY-DRIVEN RESEARCH CAPACITY-STRENGTHENING

The importance of country-driven capacity-strengthening is not a new insight. The Commission's report and many other writings have clearly recognized it. Over the years since the Commission's report, however, agencies, and particularly external agencies, have failed to sufficiently assimilate or act on this lesson. The recent messages from developing countries are also very definite, as reflected in the snapshots presented above. The first conclusion of the April 2000 WHO meeting on research capacity-strengthening captured this same view:

> *The health research agenda, including a plan for research capacity strengthening, is primarily the responsibility of the countries themselves. It was recognized that only countries could conduct a situation analysis that was relevant to local conditions and contextually accurate. Countries need to define their own research priorities and conduct locally appropriate operational research. In addition, each country needs to decide on the nature and extent of its contribution to the global research agenda. All of these principles have a direct bearing on the assessment of research capacity within a country, and on the plan and program to strengthen that capacity.*
> — WHO (2000c, pp. 7–8)

FROM A NARROW FOCUS TO A BROADER, SYSTEMS APPROACH

Most of the investment in health-research capacity, illustrated in some of the case studies above, has emphasized building the competencies of individuals, units, and institutions. Of course, these elements are important and essential, but in themselves they are not enough. The broader enabling environment in which individuals and institutions function needs more explicit attention. Although people have recognized this larger element for many years and made suggestions for creating a "research culture," the specific strategies for doing this remain elusive.

A study initiated by UNDP (Hilderbrand and Grindle 1994) gave some helpful insights concerning a systems approach to national capacity development. The study was conducted in response to a resolution of the United Nations General Assembly (Resolution 44/211), which instructed United Nations agencies to come up with a more coherent strategy for building national capacities. (The World Bank expressed similar concerns, particularly in regard to Africa [World Bank 1991].) The Harvard Institute for International Development conducted the UNDP pilot study, concentrating on public-sector capacity at the national level. It included six country case studies: Bolivia, Central African Republic, Ghana, Morocco, Sri Lanka, and Tanzania. Each case study gave a detailed analysis of national "task networks." The analysis of findings led to several important contributions, such as Dimensions of Capacity, a broad framework that goes beyond individuals and institutions to include the task networks, the public-sector context, and the national "action environment," comprising economic, political, and social factors. Based on this work, some intervention guidelines have appeared in subsequent UNDP materials (UNDP 1998). These guidelines consist of tools and models to apply at an individual, organizational, and systems levels.

SUPPLY-SIDE PREDOMINANCE

Over the past 10 years or more, something like a supply-side economic model has been the pervading mode of health-research capacity-strengthening; that is, most of the investment has gone to producing more scientists, creating stronger research units (with an optimal critical mass), and strengthening research institutions. And yet, it is widely recognized in industrialized countries that advances in science and technology are substantially driven by demand for new applications. In low-income countries, public officials, community groups, the media, and industry show a weak demand for new knowledge through research. As a result, developing countries make low investments in R&D. This leaves newly trained researchers with little incentive to remain in universities and research institutes (in part, because of low salaries); those who remain struggle hard to maintain their motivation for life-long learning and innovation. Supply-side capacity-building strategies that ignore the need to stimulate demand for research may actually further distort investment allocations (Bowles and Gintis 1996). But the strategies for stimulating demand must take account of the realities, needs, and culture of the various user groups.

It may be useful to draw a distinction between short-term problem-solving research with direct applications and longer term exploratory research; the terms *downstream* and *upstream* are sometimes used to summarize these concepts. Because the needs of low-income countries are pressing, these countries have much to gain from making significant investments in short-term problem-solving research. For some developing countries, less investment in longer term research may be appropriate. In cases in which the linkages between application-oriented research and its use are poor, even "appropriate research" may go to waste. Close links to "where the action is" will create incentives for effective research to address the pressing problems of low-income countries. Ghana gives an encouraging example of this principle (see Box 6.2).

Other chapters in this book discuss strategies for enhancing the demand and use of research by communities (Chapter 4) and policymakers (Chapter 5). To create demand is an important leadership competency for national health-research managers, as described in more detail below.

INSUFFICIENT ATTENTION TO THE EQUITY GOAL

The title of the 1990 Commission report embodied the bold idea that health research is (or should be) an "essential link to equity in development." Thankfully, in the last several years the equity goal has gradually gained more currency in the view of funders and in the work of research groups (Gwatkin 2000). Have the capacity-strengthening activities reflected this surge of interest?

In a thoughtful and forward-looking essay, written shortly after the creation of COHRED, Professor Gelia Castillo of the Philippines put forward some proposals on training researchers to pursue the equity goal (Castillo 1993). She suggested that researchers need "extra qualities," or capacities, such as those of

— Identifying, defining, and addressing the equity dimension in health and development problems;

— Comprehending and internalizing the vision that the best of science is not only in its rigour, but also in its relevance for those who have less in health;

> **Box 6.2**
>
> **Capacity development to increase demand for research in Ghana**
>
> Ghana has had a long history of health research closely linked to health services. During the 1980s, however, in part because of general economic conditions, the research-to-policy link was quite weak. In the late 1980s, an operational-research project on the feasibility of implementing a traditional birth-attendant program included a management audit at the subdistrict level. The resulting information proved to have great practical value, and it led directly to system improvement.
>
> Partly as a result of this experience, the then director of medical services established a mechanism to link research directly to the work of the Ministry of Health. His commitment to the value of research was evident in this statement: "Where I trained as a health planner, research was part of the planning process. I consider research at the operational level to be a management tool and I expect all district health managers to acquire the skill in research." Ghana created the Health Research Unit in the Ministry of Health in 1990 and published its Policy Framework on Health Research Development for the years 1992–96.
>
> Within this framework, a key strategy was building capacity at the district level to both produce and use research. This process began at the regional and provincial levels, where it created research teams and provided training, and this process now extends to district teams as well. The training includes technical aspects of research design, as well as strategies for dissemination and use of results. The management of research has gradually entered into the health-service management framework. The knowledge produced at district and regional levels has been of direct use in planning and implementing local programs. Examples include the use of Vitamin A and insecticide-treated bed nets and improvements in the use of contraceptives.
>
> More recently, Ghana adopted a revised national health-research agenda to support the key elements of the current program of health-sector reform. Thus, research focuses on issues of access and quality of health services, linkages in the health sector, health financing, and the overall effectiveness of the reform program.
>
> The Ghana experience illustrates the importance of high-level political leadership and a commitment to the use of research. It also illustrates the principle of integrating research and health-service delivery (that is, "supply" and "demand") through the creation of subnational research and action coalitions.
>
> Source: Adapted from Adjei and Gyapong (1999).

— Exposing and immersing one's self in field realities and the "facts of life" in the health system; and

— Monitoring, evaluating, and documenting the impact of health research on those for whom ENHR is supposed to make a difference.

A growing number of research initiatives are concentrating on the issue of inequities in health (as described in Chapter 2). Some of these initiatives include a capacity-development component. The World Bank has prepared a helpful guide to multicountry research programs on equity, poverty, and health (Carr et al. 1999), including a listing of projects by country.

RESEARCHERS NEED MORE THAN TECHNICAL COMPETENCE

If a major goal of health research is to enhance the health and well-being of disadvantaged populations, capacity-strengthening programs must go beyond research methodology, protocol preparation, and expertise in specialized techniques. Yet, most developing-country researchers who acquire training outside their countries will confirm that the greatest part of their training focused on these elements. Relatively little, if any, concerned the skills of advocacy, partnership development, priority-setting, facilitating the research-to-action process, or evaluating impacts. In other words, the capacity repertoire of research institutions and national health-research networks must include all aspects of the research process — from problem identification to the application of results.

The 1996 interim assessment of COHRED emphasized this point (COHRED 1996) and recommended that the elements of the ENHR process (originally identified at the 1990 Pattaya conference) be considered "technologies." In response to this recommendation, the COHRED Board created the Task Force on ENHR Competencies: the working groups in this task force have focused on specific competencies, including promotion, advocacy, and national mechanisms; priority-setting; research to action and policy; and community participation. Each group has analyzed the available experience from countries that have adopted the ENHR strategy, reviewed the relevant literature and experience from elsewhere, and prepared materials for dissemination (papers, monographs, "learning briefs," and so on). Organizations and groups, particularly country groups, are using these materials. (A list of some of these materials can be found in Chapter 8, Box 8.4.)

Furthermore, one needs to make integrated use of these competencies to address priority health and development problems at the national and subnational levels. This concept follows from some of the more recent thinking concerning the dynamics of science and research in contemporary societies. For example, in a provocative monograph entitled *The New Production of Knowledge*, Gibbons et al. (1994) described the emergence of a knowledge system known as

"Mode 2." They discussed several features of Mode-2 research: knowledge production in the context of application, social accountability, transdisciplinarity, and a diversity of organizational arrangements. Both the production and application of knowledge involve many diverse sites and "actors" — the term *social distribution* describes this feature. Success depends not only on scientific excellence but also on the usefulness (relevance) and efficiency of its mode of production. The new ICTs thus increasingly support Mode-2 activities.

STRATEGIES FOR THE FUTURE

The overall goal for the future remains unchanged. It is to ensure that all countries, particularly low-income countries, have the capacity to apply local and global knowledge to their problems in health and development (especially those of poor and disadvantaged people) and contribute to the development of global knowledge in this field. But this requires a more efficiently designed framework. This section outlines what is, to some extent, "a fresh approach" to the challenge of developing health-research capacity. The four elements of this approach are outlined below: new coalitions, new tools, new leadership, and new North–South partnerships.

NEW COALITIONS

How is it possible to create and sustain effective national health-research mechanisms and networks? The last 10 years have seen much more attention paid to this question. The underlying assumption is that many organizations and groups need to work together to strengthen the research capacities of developing countries. All these organizations and groups are stakeholders in the task of producing and using equity-oriented, priority-driven health research. But the process that leads to effective interactions among stakeholders is complex, and the participating organizations themselves need to be strong enough to contribute effectively to a national network or "system." An equally important need is to ensure that the interactions of these organizations and groups are well-coordinated and efficient.

The UNDP capacity-development study, described above (UNDP 1998), paid particular attention to national task networks (where the public sector was included). Based on a number of country case studies, UNDP specified some of the characteristics of successful national networks, including

— Policies defining goals for coordinated action;

— Specific mechanisms to facilitate frequent interaction across organizational boundaries; and

— Clarity of organizational responsibilities.

In a recent publication, the COHRED Working Group on Promotion, Advocacy and the ENHR Mechanism, reviewed and summarized the experience of several low- to middle-income countries with experience in creating or altering national mechanisms to promote ENHR (COHRED 1999). This review suggested four factors ("tough tasks") that influence the effectiveness of such mechanisms: promoting equity in health, acting as an agent for change, providing research-system support, and responding to changing circumstances. For each of these four factors, the review identified "key messages" and illustrated them with examples from low- to middle-income countries. It described several types of coalition arrangements and reported the experience of countries such as Bangladesh, Kenya, Jamaica, Nicaragua, the Philippines, South Africa, and Uganda. The snapshot from Tanzania (presented above) describes the recent creation of a Tanzanian National Health Research Forum, which has brought together all the major stakeholders in a new collaborative structure to coordinate health research.

In addition, one sees more of a focus on health-research and action coalitions at the district and subdistrict levels. Two examples illustrate this development: the Tanzania Essential Health Intervention Project (TEHIP) and the Initiative for Sub-District Support (ISDS) in South Africa.

TEHIP was established in 1997 to test innovations in evidence-based planning, priority-setting, and resource allocation at a district level (TEHIP News 1999). Consistent with Tanzania's process of health-sector reform, which features decentralization to the district level, TEHIP is conducting the project in two districts. The project is still in progress, but experience to date has confirmed that district planning coalitions can strengthen their capacities and that districts can use local evidence of various kinds in practical year-by-year decision-making and resource allocation. Ongoing research is determining the cost of this process and its impact on the burden of disease.

It is noteworthy that TEHIP takes a virtual centres-of-excellence approach, drawing on an interdisciplinary and interinstitutional consortium of Tanzanian researchers to apply their talents in addressing these practical issues. In effect, this represents a "meta-experiment" in capacity-building. As well as achieving cost-effectiveness, TEHIP has provided the additional benefit of decreasing long-standing mutual prejudices between researchers and ministry officials. Researchers learn about the realities and constraints on the health system; and government officials learn to respect the researchers' efforts to address these pressing system problems. Gradually, a climate of trust is strengthened between officials and researchers as they share data, resources, and administrative responsibilities.

Another example of the emphasis on coalitions at the district level is ISDS, which was created in 1996 to demonstrate how systematic and sustained support could improve primary health care at various sites (ISDS 1998). For example, in Mount Frere (one of the poorest districts in South Africa), ISDS established a problem-solving coalition with a clear research agenda. This involved the government health services, a local development nongovernmental organization (NGO) (Isinamva), and community members. They agreed on three research priorities: to determine who was getting sick and dying in the district and at what rate, why the death rate among children admitted to Mount Frere Hospital with malnutrition was 50%, and why drugs were not getting to the clinic shelves. All three partners participated in the community-survey design, collection of data, and analysis (McCoy 1997).

Several important lessons have emerged from the experience in the eight ISDS sites in South Africa, including the value of

— Using an initial situation-analysis exercise to establish an evidence base and to serve as a coalition-building process and;

— Having external facilitators to serve as an "honest broker";

— Tackling only a small number of common problems at any one time; and

— Using training workshops to develop and strengthen teamwork.

In essence, the new "critical mass" should be national and sub national research and learning networks focused on specific health problems and firmly linked to other relevant regional and international research efforts. These networks recognize and support various sites of knowledge generation, facilitate communication among these sites, initiate problem-oriented collaborative actions, and foster the practice of learning while doing as the model for ongoing monitoring and evaluation.

NEW TOOLS

New tools are required to ensure that health research decreases inequities in health and development. These tools should promote systems thinking to help participants in the health-research process see the whole picture, rather than component parts, and see patterns of change, rather than individual events. Examples of such tools are described below.

Tools for setting health-research priorities

The COHRED Working Group on Priority Setting has examined the experience of developing countries engaged in setting health-research priorities (COHRED–WGPS 2000). These countries have opened their priority-setting processes to several stakeholders: researchers, policymakers, health-care providers, community representatives, and sometimes funders (both national and international). Although some similarities appear across countries, each country has created its own distinctive process for determining and using priority-setting criteria. The experience to date has revealed that multistakeholder health-research priority-setting is a complex and challenging process. A frequently cited problem is moving from the identification of priorities to their actual implementation. Another is aligning the interests of external donors with stated national and local priorities. A recently published manual ("tool kit") incorporates much of the experience to date (Chongtrakul and Okello 2000).

Tools for assessing health equity

As described in Chapter 2, there is a rapidly growing interest in the issue of health inequities, and many groups are involved in designing tools and systems to describe and monitor equity in health. Most of this activity is summarized in a useful publication prepared by the World Bank (Carr et al. 1999).

Tools for monitoring resource flows

As described earlier, several countries (Malaysia, the Philippines, and Thailand) have recently undertaken studies to trace the flow of health R&D resources (COHRED 2000a). As a result of this work, COHRED is developing a training package to assist other countries in doing similar analyses.

Tools for assessing capacity development

Arising from the larger UNDP-initiated study on capacity development described earlier (Hilderbrand and Grindle 1994), ongoing work is being conducted by the Harvard Institute for International Development to develop indicators to measure investments in research capacity-strengthening. This work is addressing four levels of capacity-strengthening: individual researchers, groups, institutions, and national research communities. A progress report for this initiative was presented at the recent Annecy meeting, including a description of pilot projects currently under way to refine the indicator tools (Simon 2000).

NEW LEADERSHIP

There has been a growing interest in the role of leadership as a distinctive and important ingredient in the process of change. Some of the research and analysis of "the leadership factor" has been applied in various aspects of health-sector reform (Neufeld et al. 1995). Much of the leadership research to date, however, tends to limit itself to the private sector in industrialized countries. Nevertheless, some relevant shifts in thinking about leadership are the following:

- From thinking primarily about individual qualities to considering the specific context for leadership (in other words, less emphasis on the attributes of individual leaders and more on the leadership needed in a specific situation);
- From a focus solely on individuals to considering the importance of leadership teams (including a shift from a preoccupation with control to a focus on more participatory practices); and
- From a focus on uniformity to one on diversity, valuing differences.

Research managers in developing countries have also expressed their need for enhanced skills in research management. In response, several organizations have developed training modules and conducted seminars on this issue (IDRC and WHO 1992).

What are the special leadership competencies (both individual and collective) required to enable national health-research systems in low-income countries to reduce health inequities? This section proposes some of these special competencies in addition to the general attributes required for any leadership, such as the ability to articulate a collective vision, inspire, and "seize the day."

Knowledge management

There is an increasing emphasis on the importance of the "knowledge economy" in economic and social development (World Bank 1999). What does this mean for health-research managers in low-income countries? Given the remarkable progress in the development and use of ICTs, potentially all countries should have ready access to a global knowledge base. More specifically, health-research managers should be able to apply all the available knowledge, both local and global, to specific local health problems. But the transaction costs of communication are high in low-income countries. The reasons for this include poor communication infrastructures and limited access to global knowledge sources. Busy health managers in low-income countries are often also doing work that in industrialized countries would be that of support staff and have little time and even less opportunity to acquire the necessary skills and habits to use ICTs.

Given the potential of the available ICTs, a special opportunity currently presents itself to the global health-research community — an opportunity for international agencies and partners in the North to facilitate the development of the knowledge management capacities of health-research managers in the South. There are several encouraging examples of agencies responding to this opportunity. One is the Scientists for Health and Research for Development project. This project has developed an interactive Web-based system for storing and accessing information concerning research projects, funding agencies, networks, and research documentation (for more information, visit http://www.shared.de/). Another is the Health Information for Development project, launched in January 2000; it is preparing a global directory of Health Information Resource Centres, among its other activities (see http://www.iswp.org).

In addition to needing the skills to use ICTs, knowledge managers must also be able to critically appraise the validity of the evidence base for health interventions and interpret it for appropriate application. The Cochrane Collaboration is an international coalition of clinicians and consumers working mainly through the Internet to design, conduct, report, disseminate, and criticize systematic reviews in all areas of health care (more information is available at http://www.hiru.mcmaster.ca/cochrane).

Creating demand

As noted earlier, efforts to build research capacity have had a preoccupation with the supply side and paid insufficient attention to fostering a demand for research. What does this mean in terms of specific competencies for health-research leadership in developing countries? Stimulating a demand for research may mean targeting user groups more than researchers. User groups may include legislators, the media, district development committees, and the private sector. In South Africa, for example, national legislators helped in designing a country-wide survey of health facilities, including a mechanism to monitor progress in provision of equitable services (HST 2000).

Coalition-building

If research and learning networks and coalitions are to become an increasingly important feature of national health-research systems, this can be expected to create greater demand for coalition-building skills. These skills are particularly important in developing countries, where intersectoral collaboration is required for research and effective action on most health problems. Several important analyses of intersectoral collaboration are available, and they offer insights into the role of facilitators in collaboration ("coalition-builders") (Harris 1995; Burdach 1998).

Developing leadership

All too often, new health-research managers and management teams find themselves unprepared to meet the responsibilities they are taking on. Typically, senior researchers are thrust into leadership positions based primarily on seniority and past scientific or academic performance. Although some managers already use informal methods to prepare future leaders, it would be useful to pay more attention to specific strategies for developing leadership. These may include a program of reading and discussion on effective leadership, explicit succession planning, and systematic mentoring (Pegg 1999).

NEW NORTH–SOUTH PARTNERSHIPS

Despite the good intentions of developing countries in creating and maintaining self-sustaining health-research systems, the fact remains that many highly depend on resources from the North. This applies to the support of health-sector reform generally and to health-research activities within the health sector. The reality is that North–South interactions will remain an important feature of health research in many developing countries for the foreseeable future. How well do these partnerships contribute to strengthening national health-research capacities in low-income countries? What can be learned in this regard from the experience of the past 10 years?

Some insights into these questions are available in the recent self-assessments of some bilateral agencies. In a thoughtful compilation of essays, the Swedish Agency for Research Cooperation with Developing Countries (SAREC) reviewed its experience of 20 years (SAREC 1995). A focus on strengthening the capacities of university departments has been a particular feature of the support for research (including health research) offered by SAREC (now the Swedish International Development Cooperation Agency [SIDA] – SAREC). Its strategy for the 1990s was to continue with this emphasis, but with the additional element of measures to support the university as a whole, including research training and university administration. It began using an increasing share of the total allocation to strengthen the conditions for research at the universities, such as support for reforms, research management, libraries, Internet connectivity, and laboratories. A relatively new feature, at that time, was the contribution to university funds for research, which was intended to stimulate systems for peer review and decision-making on research. The concluding essay summarized the overall thrust of this volume: "research and researchers should play an active and proactive role in the process of change. This may be at variance with a more traditional view of the researcher as an 'objective' and detached scholar, whose hands should not be tainted by personal participation in actual events" (SAREC 1995, p. 187). Current SIDA–SAREC policies and programs are described in a more recent publication (SIDA–SAREC 2000).

In 1997, Norway's Ministry of Foreign Affairs commissioned a comprehensive study of institutional development in Norwegian bilateral assistance, examining the experience of three development-assistance channels used by the Norwegian Agency for International Development (NAID): the public sector, private commercial firms, and NGOs (GON 1998). The report found that in general there was an increasing awareness and commitment to institutional development (capacity development) among public institutions and NGOs. It found, however, that policy objectives were unclear, that overall development perspectives were missing, and that the empirical base for assessing results was weak. It put forward a comprehensive set of recommendations with application at three levels: the Ministry of Foreign Affairs, NAID, and Norwegian organizations. The recommendations for the latter included putting "a stronger emphasis on developing competence and capacity for problem-solving in developing countries" (GON 1998, p. 49), that is, on the capacity for learning.

In the Netherlands, the Directorate General for International Cooperation developed a "demand-driven, research cooperation programme for health in Africa" (Wolffers et al. 1998, p. 1654). This initiative focused on three countries: Benin, Ghana, and Mozambique. The first phase of this exploration found that "conventional research cooperation is often counterproductive for development of a sustainable research environment" (Wolffers et al. 1998, p. 1654). This initiative has led to a cooperative health-research program involving Ghana and the Netherlands, which genuinely attempts to "put Southern requirements first" (Wolffers et al. 1998, p. 1653). It will be important to monitor this and similar experiments and to continue to disseminate the lessons learned to the global health-research community.

Multilateral agencies, too, have reviewed their role in capacity development at the country level. WHO recently conducted a review of its contributions (Lucas et al. 1997). On national capacity for managing health services, the report found that top management is often unstable, with high turnover rates of senior officials (such as Ministers of Health and professional and administrative heads). Although the study did not specifically examine the issue of national health-research capacity, it did review the development of health services more generally and recommended a new approach, which the investigators named "the essential presence," tailoring WHO's contribution to the needs and capacity of individual countries and to the contributions of other external agencies. The principle author of the report later called on WHO to improve its own analytic capacity to adequately function in this new mode (Lucas 1998).

With the recent creation of the Department of Research Policy and Cooperation (described in Chapter 1), WHO is assigning higher priority to health research in its profile of work. Importantly, the challenge of research capacity-strengthening has been a major focus of attention of this new department. Evidence of this is the consultative process of the Relevant Research Excellence Accelerates Complete Health initiative, with its emphasis on promoting a new paradigm for research capacity-strengthening. The criteria for the International Health Research Awards (to be presented at the October 2000 conference in Bangkok) also reflect this invitation to innovate. Similarly, the April 2000 meeting in Annecy had some welcome features signaling a new beginning (WHO 2000c). Although initiated by WHO, this meeting was cosponsored by several other groups. Most of the participants were from developing countries. It gave the highest priority to in-depth discussions among "working teams" to analyze country experiences, integrate other inputs into the context of country realities, and put forward "action ideas." The outputs of the meeting consisted of two sets of conclusions: a description of "key strategies and principles" for research capacity-strengthening; and "action ideas" to be assimilated into WHO's new framework and vision for research capacity-strengthening.

A recent special issue of the journal *Health Policy and Planning* examined the question of coordination and management of external resources in the health sectors of low-income countries; it included several country case studies (Walt et al. 1999b). Much of this analysis derived from projects funded through loans from the major development banks. Although the focus was not specifically on the production and use of health research, some important insights from the analysis are applicable to the issue of North–South partnerships. They include the importance of both formal and informal relationships and the inherent instability of the process of managing external resources. It also stressed the importance of paying particular attention to the context-specific conditions of each country.

A helpful description of important principles of North–South partnerships for research appears in a recent publication of the Swiss Commission for Research Partnerships with Developing Countries (SCRPDC 1998). These principles are summarized in Box 6.3.

CONCLUSION

The American poet Robert Frost once wrote, "I have promises to keep; and miles to go before I sleep." So it is with the hopes and prospects for health-research capacity-strengthening articulated 10 years ago. At best, progress in the intervening decade has been modest. To more effectively build a national capacity for equity-oriented health research, we will need to make dramatic shifts in our conceptualization of the challenge and take steps to meet it. Current supply-side strategies too often reinforce the prevailing market and peer incentives that focus research on the problems of the rich. In fact, the predominant international emphasis on new-product development can work against equity.

We need to make a major shift to demand-driven capacity development, taking guidance from the needs and realities of developing countries. National leaders should have support for their efforts to forge problem-oriented research and learning coalitions and networks. It will be important to develop and apply new purpose-specific tools. To exploit the promise of the information-technology

> **Box 6.3**
>
> ## The 11 Principles of Research Partnership
>
> Included are illustrative questions adapted from a "checklist" for each principle.
>
> 1. Decide on the objectives together
>   — Did all the relevant actors and people who will be affected by the research participate in developing the theme of the research?
> 2. Build up mutual trust
>   — Do all the partners know each other well enough, and do they trust each other?
> 3. Share information; develop networks
>   — Has provision been made on both organizational and technical levels for all the partners to have sufficient regular contact with each other?
> 4. Share responsibility
>   — Will all the responsible partners see all the documents relevant to them?
> 5. Create transparency
>   — Are there clear and fair rules about who has the authority to make what decisions?
> 6. Monitor and evaluate the collaboration
>   — Have the criteria for internal evaluation been jointly defined and are they known?
> 7. Disseminate the results
>   — Are there plans for passing on project results to the people directly affected?
> 8. Apply the results
>   — Will all those concerned take part in plans to put the results into practice?
> 9. Share profits equitably
>   — Will all the partners be considered when the results of the research are published?
> 10. Increase research capacity
>   — Will the collaboration contribute to increasing scientific capacity of all partners?
> 11. Build on the achievements
>   — Will the research results increase awareness of the importance of research?
>
>   Source: SCRPDC (1998, excerpts from pp. 15–34).

revolution, strategies will be needed to reduce the costs of communication for research producers and users in low-income countries. And leaders in research in both the North and the South must strengthen their capacities to participate effectively in truly collaborative partnerships, based on mutual respect and shared goals.

CHAPTER 7

REGIONAL PERSPECTIVES

*Javid Hashmi, Tamas Koos, Peter Makara, Abdelhay Mechbal,
Mutuma Mugambi, Victor Neufeld, Alberto Pellegrini Filho, David Picou,
and Chitr Sitthi-amorn*

SUMMARY

This chapter explores the link between national health-research activities and regional organizations. The analysis covers six regions where most countries are in the low- to middle-income range. Research leaders from these regions provide profiles ("snapshots") of the regions — past, present, and future — and describe existing organizations, in particular those that influence health research at the national level. This chapter also discusses lessons learned and future possibilities.

AFRICA

Historical records show that centuries ago, Africa was a strong contributor to science in such areas as advanced mathematics, astronomy, agriculture, medicine, and other fields. During the colonial period, health research focused largely on conditions affecting expatriates and was based in topic-specific research centres. With independence, countries took over these existing research structures and, together with universities, tried to revise health-research systems to meet the countries' needs.

Over the past 10 years, 24 African countries have adopted the Essential National Health Research (ENHR) strategy, identifying national health-research priorities, strengthening coordination mechanisms, and promoting networking. Regional structures include the African ENHR network, the World Health Organization (WHO) regional system, and a number of other health and health-research networks. Overall, there is a sense that, collectively, the networks have not significantly strengthened national health-research systems. Out of the lessons and experiences of the past, African countries have developed a vision and agenda for health research for the future: health research must be country-driven, with a particular emphasis on research that places equity at the forefront of health development.

ASIA

More than half of the world's people live in Asia, a region of remarkable diversity of every kind — economic, cultural, social, and political. WHO allocates the countries of Asia to three regional offices. Several networks and organizations are concerned with health research, both within countries and in the region as a whole. Organizations, such as the Tropical Medicine and Public Health Center of the Southeast Asian Ministers of Education Organization (SEAMEO–TROPMED), have made important contributions to health research, including research capacity-strengthening. However, with some exceptions, regional organizations have been slow to foster research cooperation on new and emerging health issues. More can be done to create and facilitate intercountry research coalitions to address problems such as the impact of trade liberalization on health services and the effects of human migration on the transfer of health risks. The section on Asia describes a recent experience involving the creation of the Asian Forum for Health Research. It has focused on the specific issue of preparing an "Asian voice" for the October 2000 conference on health research and has innovatively and effectively engaged the energy and contributions of many national and regional health-research groups.

THE CARIBBEAN

The section on the Caribbean presents the experience of this region's English- and Dutch-speaking islands. Relevant regional structures are the Conference of Ministers Responsible for Health (CMRH), the Pan American Health Organization (PAHO), and the Caribbean Health Research Council (CHRC). Analyses of papers submitted and presented to the annual scientific meetings of the CHRC indicate a gradual shift in the content of research toward health problems that health ministers have designated the highest priorities for the region. Overall, however, a "research culture" is lacking in the region, which has low levels of government support for health research and a fairly weak capacity in terms of infrastructure, management, and links to health policy. Countries perceive CHRC as making some strong contributions, such as a forum (the annual scientific meeting) and training workshops, administration of research grants, and advocacy of the ENHR strategy. Four countries in this group now have ENHR committees, and a recent initiative is under way to identify regional health-research priorities.

CENTRAL AND EASTERN EUROPEAN COUNTRIES AND NEWLY INDEPENDENT STATES

There is a strong tradition of health-related research in the Central and Eastern European countries and newly independent states (former Soviet Union) (CEEC–NIS), which has world-renowned scientists and research institutions. With the dramatic socioeconomic transitions of the late 1980s and early 1990s, the region suffered a concurrent drop in research funding and a decline in research capacity in many countries. Rapid social change created new challenges for health researchers, particularly in behavioural research (research on social inequalities) and health-systems research. During this period, many of the previous regional structures disintegrated, but new relationships were created, particularly with counterparts in the industrialized countries of Western Europe. New regional networks have been appearing, such as the Central Asian Research Information Network (CARIN), initiated by the WHO's Regional Office for Europe. Despite these major system changes of the past decade, many health-research institutions have survived — a tribute to the strong legacy of human resources and research traditions. Now the challenge is to build on this base and strengthen capacities in such areas as priority-setting, research management, community participation, and mutually beneficial coalition-building.

EASTERN MEDITERRANEAN

The 23 countries under the purview of WHO's Regional Office for the Eastern Mediterranean show a remarkable diversity. Old civilizations and entrenched cultural traditions are characteristic of this region. Although its diversity is reflected in the status of health research across countries, some general features pertain to most countries: the planners' demand for research is minimal; for the most part, only the researchers establish research priorities; few countries have national health-research networks; and research capacities are weak, particularly in the broader aspects of the research process. The only regional health-research structures are those facilitated by WHO's regional office. A regional task force on health research, established in 1986, has assisted a number of countries in developing national health-research policies and strategies. Few countries in the region have adopted the ENHR strategy. A recent regional consultation emphasized the importance of multistakeholder national health-research organizations and the need for a regional health-research forum.

Three general conclusions can be drawn from the regional analysis:

— Regional health-research structures should primarily respond to country needs;

— Regional organizations are most effective if they provide distinctive added value, over and above what countries can and should do for themselves; and

— Several regions see the need to create and strengthen regional health-research forums to fulfill special functions, such as advocacy of the perspectives and needs of countries in global discussions.

LATIN AMERICA

The profile of science and technology (S&T) in Latin America during the 1990s reflects its general recovery from the financial crisis of the previous decade. As a result, the region has seen increases in health research and development (R&D) investment, the number of researchers, and the volume of scientific publications. Most of these increases occurred in a small number of countries — principally Argentina, Brazil, Chile, and Mexico. Regional health trends feature decreasing mortality rates and increased life expectancy, on one hand, but widening health inequities, on the other. The Latin American health-research community is trying to respond to this changing situation by increasing the emphasis on health-research priority-setting and paying more attention to the dissemination and use of research results. PAHO has concentrated particularly on the health-research needs of low-income countries in the region, promoting institutional networks to conduct research on high-priority problems. Several of these coalitions focus on health inequities. Among the lessons learned is the realization that the change process is difficult and slow — for example, the use by scientific councils of a broader set of criteria in the peer-review process, including policy relevance. The coalitions are using the new information and communication technologies (ICTs) to support more decentralized, participatory, and problem-oriented research policies and practices.

INTRODUCTION

For many countries, health-research activities are substantially influenced by interactions with other countries, facilitated by regional structures and arrangements. These arrangements range in nature from informal networks to formal organizations. Sometimes they are geographic subdivisions of global organizations, such as the WHO regional offices. Potentially, countries benefit from these regional affiliations through information exchange, funding, technical support, and participation in a range of collaborative intercountry projects and activities.

This chapter explores the relationship between regional structures and national health-research activities, including analyses of six regions: Africa, Asia, the Caribbean, Central and Eastern Europe, Eastern Mediterranean, and Latin America. Mostly low- to middle-income countries are found in these regions.

Research leaders from these six regions provide profiles (snapshots) of their regions, outlining the main developments over the past 10 years or more, the current situation, and future trends. They describe regional organizations that influence national health-research activities and comment on how regional arrangements have helped (or possibly hindered) national efforts to conduct equity-oriented, priority-driven health research. In some cases, they discuss lessons learned and make suggestions for the future. A summary of some crosscutting issues and observations concludes the chapter.

AFRICA

HISTORICAL BACKGROUND

People often have the false impression that Africa has lacked a tradition of S&T. Yet, history tells that people in various parts of the continent made studies and practical use of advanced mathematics, astronomy, steel-engineering, architecture, agriculture, and medicine. European explorers and colonizers divided the continent into spheres of political and economic influence, and this has had a profound impact on the direction of general development. It also appears to have erased past scientific achievements and blocked further progress.

During occupation, the interests of colonial governments largely determined investments in science. They gave priority in research to areas of direct commercial value, such as agriculture and livestock development. Health research was a low priority, except in the case of diseases posing a threat to empire-building. With this end, the earliest of the research institutes were contracted to expatriate scientists from colonizing-country medical-research councils, institutes, and universities. The original research laboratories were therefore led by such bodies as the British Medical Research Council, the Institute Pasteur, and schools of tropical medicine in London, Liverpool, and Antwerp.

Colonial governments invested in health research to varying extents, from minimal inputs to extensive regional networks of laboratories. In the early stages, research and control programs targeted such health issues as malaria and other tropical diseases, hemorrhagic fevers, and a few uncommon conditions. The African-based laboratories, in collaboration with parent institutions, made significant scientific contributions in the epidemiology, etiology, transmission, and management of tropical parasitic diseases. Many young visiting research scientists made their careers in these laboratories; some became world authorities in tropical health.

Before independence, the region developed a few strong health-research networks. The East African Medical Research Council, in the former British Empire, ran a chain of laboratories in Kenya, Uganda, and Tanzania, each with specialized functions. In French West Africa, research was undertaken in networks supervised by the Scientific Research Institute for Development, the French Institute for Black Africa, and the Institute Pasteur. These networks were well established in many countries, including Benin, Burkina Faso, Cameroon, and Guinea–Conakry. South Africa, as an isolated country, set up its own South African Institute for Medical Research, although for the most part the growing mining industry determined its initial interests. Even though these institutions conducted high-quality research, they gave little priority to developing indigenous research capacities.

With independence and the departure of expatriate scientists, some laboratories, especially in the former French countries, were abandoned. Often these laboratories were left in the hands of technicians who lacked research-leadership abilities. Thus, each country, as it gained statehood, inherited whatever research structures were in existence. Lacking a research culture, most countries paid little attention to locally directed S&T development. In the early stages, they emphasized the adoption of technologies available on the market. Development and direction of health research were largely left in the hands of emerging local universities, which, in collaboration with their external partners, set the priority agenda. Not surprisingly, individuals, institutions, and funding agencies drove the priorities.

With increasing recognition of the value of research in development, countries in the region began to place science and research on a higher platform, and they established research councils and ministries of S&T. Unfortunately, policy decisions did not always translate into effective implementation. Often, they failed to provide commensurate funding for research to councils, institutes, and universities, and this stifled outputs. Within the total scientific scenario, health research has traditionally received low priority. Typically, government leaders have regarded funding for the social sector, including health, as a financial burden, rather than as an investment.

At the start of the new millennium, Africa's contribution to the global S&T portfolio is marginal, with the continent's share of the world's scientific output having fallen to 0.3%. Furthermore, sub-Sahara Africa hardly benefits from 1% of the global health-research expenditure. Such low investments in health research and the prevalence of demotivating environments have resulted in a low capacity for research and the flight of human capital. In the mean time, many countries have been spending large sums on external consultants and technical assistance, expenditures that currently consume nearly 40% of overseas development assistance.

Despite the prevailing challenges of new and reemerging diseases, increasing health inequalities, and the impacts of globalization, hope is mounting. The past few years have shown signs of better governance and improving economies, both of which may direct more resources to health and health research.

REGIONAL NETWORKS

Since the 1990 report of the Commission on Health Research for Development 24 African countries, with the assistance of the Council on Health Research for Development (COHRED), have adopted the ENHR strategy. Although not all of these countries have successfully implemented their plans, nearly half have made major strides in revisiting their national health-research systems. Priority-setting has been at the forefront in determining a new approach to research development. In an inclusive way, countries have analyzed health situations and the status of health research, organized district and regional consultations, and held national workshops for multiple stakeholders to determine a priority agenda to drive future research. Another major outcome of these consultations has been discussions on national research mechanisms to advocate research and promote networking. A few countries have evolved fairly sophisticated mechanisms. On the downside, as a result of shortages of local and external funding, countries have faced difficulties in translating priorities into research projects.

At the regional level, the African ENHR network started in 1994 and has identified a "focal point" (coordinator). In 1996, the network hosted 11 other regional health-research networks in an attempt to forge closer collaboration between them. As a result of one of the recommendations, African Research Organizations and Networks started operations to enhance electronic dialogue between health researchers in the region. Since then network meetings have taken place annually. These meetings have provided a useful forum for sharing country experiences and developing work plans. Promotion efforts have enlarged the network, and a number of countries have now produced detailed monographs. Country studies on, for example, capacity development, community participation, and priority-setting have been commissioned, and findings have been used to guide country research processes. Stronger countries have continued to support the weaker ones. A major achievement of the African ENHR network has been its facilitation of the African consultation to prepare for the conference in Bangkok in October 2000.

Forty-six African countries are members of the WHO regional system, and each has a WHO representative. Health Ministers meet regularly as a regional committee and focus deliberations on health strategies for the region. Although the WHO regional office has a research agenda, it has so far not been particularly proactive in health-research development. The Organization of African Unity, which also has an S&T desk, has not been a significant player in health research. (These two regional bodies nevertheless have the potential for leadership in health research.) Apart from the African ENHR network, other major research networks with some history in the region include the following:

— Commonwealth Regional Health Community;

— Joint Project on Health Systems Research (now under the WHO regional office);

— International Clinical Epidemiology Network;

— International Health Policy Programme;

— Network of Public Health Institutions;

— Social Science and Medicine Africa Network;

— University Partnerships Project; and

— African Network on Malaria and Vaccine Trials.

The African region has many other recently formed networks.

Many respondents in the African consultation believed that regional networks can serve a useful role as catalysts for research development in the region. However, the widespread opinion was that the existing networks have not collaborated well and that this is why they have not made the expected impacts, particularly in capacity-building, collaborative research, and information exchange. In the opinion of many, the majority of these networks lack a broader vision of Africa's health-research needs and consequently have tended to operate in pursuit of narrow interests. The last 10 years have witnessed the formation of a number of international initiatives, all aimed at supporting health research in developing countries. Some of these are COHRED, the Global Forum for Health Research, the Alliance for Policy and Health Systems Research, and Scientists for Health and Research for Development.

Both regional and international networks have, without doubt, made contributions within their specific mandates; in particular, most have provided training, organized meetings and conferences for research dissemination, brought policymakers and researchers closer together, and enhanced collaboration. However, there is a widespread feeling that they have made, collectively, no significant impact. They have not given priority to issues profoundly affecting the development of health research, such as policy, operational mechanisms, funding, networking, information technology, ethics, and partnership arrangements. The narrow territorial interests of some of the networks may even have contributed to further fragmentation of research.

PROSPECTS FOR THE FUTURE

Out of the past lessons and experiences, African countries have developed a vision and agenda for health research in the coming decades. Particular emphasis will be on research that places equity at the forefront of health development. The way ahead for health research at the national level is very country specific. However, in all cases, health research must be country driven. Other efforts, whether regional or global, must support that principle. Greatest attention must be directed to capacity development, coordination, and the enabling environment. Capacity-building will be broad and will relate to quantity and quality, multidisciplinary research, demand for and use of research, health leadership and management for research, policy analysis, publication and dissemination, partnership development, communication technology, and institutional facilities. All countries see an important need for an efficient national coordination mechanism. Whatever the mechanism, it should be widely accepted and have political and financial support from government and other national partners. It should be appropriate to the country, co-owned, transparent, and bottom up, with a clear orientation toward national and district problems. A national forum is worth considering, as already exemplified in a few countries. Among its functions should be advocacy, coordination, networking, and knowledge use.

At the regional level, it is strongly believed that Africa should have an effective, autonomous health-research forum, with a secretariat. The forum should be located in Africa, have a board of directors, and work in close association with the WHO regional office and other major partners in health-research development. The main functions of this mechanism would be to define general policy and work plans for the region, serve as an "African voice" to speak for Africa in its dealings with international initiatives and development partners, provide active networking, act as a support mechanism for country activities, perform analytical functions, and provide oversight on generic concerns of ethics, good practices in North–South collaboration, and mobilization of funds.

At the global level, there is concern that most of the international initiatives do not seriously represent the interests of Africans. The fragmentation at the international level leads to confusion in national research systems: arbitrary choices concerning what to do, who to collaborate with, and who to bring in as experts. People in most countries resent this mode of operation. Their wish is to see a more united donor community that respects national priorities and mechanisms and works in partnership to promote better management, greater effectiveness, and more sustainable research. They want to see a further strengthening of the model that COHRED sets, with its focus on national research mechanisms.

ASIA

It is virtually impossible, in a few paragraphs, to present an accurate picture of this vast part of the world. More than 50% of the world's people live in Asia, and the region shows large variations of every kind (economic, cultural, social, and political) between and within countries. India alone is said to have 40 distinct language groups; some Indian states have populations approaching 100 million people.

Within the continent of Asia are subregions that differ markedly from each other.

Added to this remarkable diversity is the effect of globalization. A striking instance is the recent economic crisis, with its unexpected and serious impacts, not only on those Southeast Asian countries directly affected, but also on economies around the world. With the loosening of trade restrictions, the health sector has seen a rapid growth in private medical services, medical technology, and uncontrolled health-insurance markets, which, in some instances, have led to wider health disparities (COHRED 2000a).

REGIONAL STRUCTURES

Several distinct trade and economic organizations operate within Asia, such as the Association of Southeast Asian Nations (ASEAN) and the South Asian Association for Regional Cooperation. The WHO system allocates Asian countries to three regions. Countries such as Afghanistan and Pakistan come under the purview of the WHO Regional Office for the Eastern Mediterranean. The rest of Asia is divided between the regional offices for Southeast Asia and for the Western Pacific. Other global agencies divide Asia into various constellations.

Many health-research structures and organizations work within the larger Asian region. Vast countries, such as China and India, have their own large health-research organizations and networks. For example, the Indian Council for Medical Research comprises a network of problem-specific research centres scattered throughout the country; it serves as a strong coordinating mechanism for health research in this country of now 1 billion people. A Chinese example is the China Network for Training and Research in Health Economics and Financing. Created under the auspices of the Ministry of Health, this network comprises the China National Health Economics Institute and 10 other institutions located in medical universities throughout the country.

Some regional health-research organizations have been in existence for many years; an example is SEAMEO–TROPMED — an organization devoted to the support of health development, including health research, in Southeast Asia. (See Chapter 6 for a more detailed description of SEAMEO–TROPMED activities.) Other groups are more recent — an example is the Southeast Asia Clinical Epidemiology Network (SEACLEN). Led by training centres in Indonesia, the Philippines, and Thailand, SEACLEN is an active network of academic professionals with expertise in clinical epidemiology and public-health research. Other examples are the recently created Asia–Pacific Health Economics Network and the Asia–Pacific Network of the International Forum for Social Sciences and Health.

IMPACT OF REGIONAL ARRANGEMENTS ON NATIONAL HEALTH RESEARCH

Regional organizations such as SEAMEO–TROPMED have spearheaded investments in health research. In some areas, regional and global investments have been complementary. For example, both SEAMEO–TROPMED and the global Special Programme for Research and Training in Tropical Diseases (TDR) have contributed to direct research and capacity-strengthening; this has been instrumental in improving health and decreasing the incidence of infectious disease.

The WHO regional offices have made useful contributions to national efforts by fostering exchanges between countries and, in some instances, stimulating intercountry research collaboration. Collaboration between WHO regions is increasing but needs further development. Collaborative activities sponsored by regional trade and economic organizations (such as ASEAN) have contributed some benefits in the health sector and, indirectly, in the health research of participating countries.

Regional organizations, however, have been slow to use their strengths in fostering research cooperation on new and emerging health and development problems. A recent encouraging example is the network for Surveillance of Infectious Diseases operating among countries in the Mekong Basin; partial assistance from the Rockefeller Foundation is helping to establish this network. Regional research cooperation would be helpful in resolving such problems as the following:

— Health disparities resulting from privatization of health insurance and health services, as a consequence of trade liberalization;

— Impact of human migration on the transfer of health risks, such as epidemics of infectious diseases like AIDS and zoonoses (for example, the spread of chicken and Nippah viruses);

— Rising cost of health care, as a result of chronic and social diseases, such as drug dependence, sexually transmitted diseases, injuries, and mental illness; and

— Global environmental impacts on human health in the region, such as land degradation, persistent use of organic pollutants, and increasing traffic congestion.

Regional health-research networks and organizations can also assist countries with some of the more difficult aspects of strengthening national health-research systems. Some possible forms of assistance would be the following:

— Convincing decision-makers (in government and in the private sector) that funding for health research can be a sound economic and social investment, not just a marginal budget item (countries in the region need stronger strategies to link national health services, including health policy, and national health-research systems); and

— Broadening the base of stakeholders in the health-research process to include citizens and nongovernmental organizations (NGOs). Health research can empower citizens to make good choices and thus participate in policy processes. Health research can also make NGOs more effective. Citizens and NGOs can in turn demand accountability from governments and health-research organizations and serve as a check and balance on governance, encouraging international donors to focus on country priorities.

LESSONS LEARNED

Some useful and important lessons can be learned from recent experience with a health-research network in Asia — a mechanism that became known as the Asian Forum for Health Research. A number of regional health-research leaders saw the need for health-research groups in Asia to prepare for the October 2000 conference. An ad hoc planning group convened in September 1999. It comprised representatives from several health research networks and organizations, the WHO regional offices, and various countries. The group decided to use a three-stage, innovative participatory strategy to engage a wide range of stakeholders: a preforum dialogue, 3-day forum, and postforum follow-up arrangements leading to the October 2000 conference. A 5-month preconference electronic dialogue involved 300 individuals across Asia. Among its aims were sharing information and determining key research issues of relevance to the Asian region, for further discussion at the forum.

About 100 people met for the 3-day forum in Manila in February 2000. The format of this meeting included some innovations, such as plenary roundtable discussions, collaborative team discussion of regional research priorities, a marketplace (including a "speaker's corner"), and a technology-support centre. An outcome of the forum was a draft of an Asian-voice statement. This synthesis document captured the key ideas and recommendations from the working teams, with a view to taking them forward to the international meeting in Bangkok (Sitthi-amorn 2000[1]). Following the meeting in Manila, the participants used a website to continue their exchange of information and dialogue. Organizers agreed to expand the network by encouraging each of the original 300 dialogue participants to invite others from their own institutions and countries.

The Asian-forum participants and planners have reflected on the lessons learned through this process, including the following:

— By focusing on a specific issue (in this case, the need to prepare an Asian voice for the upcoming conference), it was possible to engage the interest, energy, and commitment of many national and regional health-research groups;

— Electronic communication proved to be a satisfactory and efficient method of facilitating the participation of 300 individuals across Asia; and

— A small coordinating team (supported by some technical expertise) required considerable effort to facilitate the electronic dialogue, plan and manage the actual forum activities, and sustain the follow-up planning.

THE CARIBBEAN

For the purposes of this section, *the Caribbean* means the English-speaking Caribbean, made up of 18 countries and territories where English is the first language,[2] and the 5 Dutch-speaking islands of the Netherlands Antilles.[3] They are set in a sea of islands spanning about 3 500 km between Belize and Guyana. These countries show wide

---

[1] Sitthi-amorn, C. 2000. Report of the Asian Forum for Health Research. Manila, the Philippines, 17–19 Feb 2000. Internet: http://161.200.33.29. (In draft.)

[2] Antigua and Barbuda, Anguilla, the Bahamas, Barbados, Belize, Bermuda, British Virgin Islands, Cayman Islands, Dominica, Grenada, Guyana, Jamaica, Montserrat, St Kitts-Nevis, St Lucia, St Vincent and the Grenadines, Trinidad and Tobago, and the Turks and Caicos.

[3] Bonaire, Curaçao, Saba, St Eustatius, and St Martin.

variations in size and population, resources and capabilities, religions and cultures, and ethnic groups. The English-speaking Caribbean has a combined population of about 6 million, and the Netherlands Antilles has a population of 200 000.

By the mid-1970s, the global economic crisis threatened to erode gains made in health conditions in the region. Infrastructure was deteriorating, supplies were dwindling, and many health personnel were migrating to high-income countries. It was unlikely that the strategy of national self-reliance would, by itself, correct the decline and restore the previous rate of improvement in health conditions.

REGIONAL STRUCTURES AND ARRANGEMENTS

Health services

In 1986, CMRH adopted six priority health areas, under the Caribbean Cooperation in Health (CCH) initiative: environmental protection (including vector control), human-resource development, chronic noncommunicable illnesses and accidents, strengthening health systems, food and nutrition, and maternal and child health and population activities. In 1988, CMRH added AIDS to the list. An assessment of this initiative in 1992–94 found it was beneficial to the Caribbean countries.

In 1996, CMRH mandated a redefinition of the CCH initiative for 1997–2001. It held a regional consultation in 1997 with people from a wide range of disciplines, and it then selected eight priority health areas, recommended strategies for implementation, and identified areas for joint action. The new priorities were health-systems development, human-resource development, family health, food and nutrition, chronic noncommunicable illnesses, communicable diseases, mental health, and environmental health.

Caribbean Health Research Council

The English-speaking governments of the region have supported CHRC as a regional organization, which until 1997 was known as the Commonwealth Caribbean Medical Research Council. Over the past 45 years, it has had major responsibility for promoting health research. Its activities have included

— Promoting and supporting the establishment of ENHR by helping countries define national health-research priorities and create national ENHR committees (to date, four countries have these committees: Barbados, Curaçao, Jamaica, and Trinidad and Tobago);

- Organizing annual scientific meetings, including an annual symposium;
- Administering a block-grant scheme; and
- Strengthening research capacity through a program of research-skills workshops.

Pan American Health Organization

PAHO has a representative in most Caribbean countries and also has an office in Barbados for the Caribbean program coordinator; the office houses PAHO staff specifically assigned to areas such as chronic noncommunicable illnesses and maternal and child health. It is one of the most important regional organizations in health and health research in the Caribbean and has taken the lead role in producing CCH I and CCH II, the publication *Health Status of the Caribbean,* and several other documents. PAHO facilitates health research by mobilizing resources, convening meetings and workshops, and arranging technical-cooperation activities. PAHO works for and through national governments and collaborates with other regional organizations to improve health.

PROFILE OF HEALTH RESEARCH IN THE CARIBBEAN

The Caribbean has six medical schools, including three affiliated with the University of the West Indies, and these schools conduct research to varying degrees. The region has nine health-research institutions, which focus on subjects ranging from human nutrition, to chronic noncommunicable illnesses, to environmental health. CHRC and PAHO also support, facilitate, and coordinate research across the region.

The topics of the papers at the annual scientific meetings reflect the content of health research in the region. Content analyses of these papers were conducted in 1995 and 2000. The 1995 survey showed a gradual increase in health-service research to 40% of all papers by 1994 (over more than two decades) and a decrease in laboratory studies to about 20% (Walrond 1995). Clinical studies remained about the same (25%), as did those in epidemiology and public health (10–15%). The survey conducted in 2000 was done to determine the degree to which research activities matched the eight regional health priorities (Picou 2000). About half of the papers presented before 1984 related to health-service priorities; since then the proportion has increased to 60%.

One can infer some indication of the status of the health-research system itself from recent surveys in Jamaica and Trinidad. These surveys indicate that the main features of the health-research system in the Caribbean are as follows:

- Individual researchers drive and finance a significant proportion of research;
- Universities and health-research institutions do the majority of research;
- Less than half of completed research appears in peer-reviewed journals;
- Governments commission or conduct only a small proportion of research;
- Researchers perceive constraints such as
  - Inadequate funding, time, equipment, and facilities,
  - Problems with data collection and analysis, and
  - Lack of support staff; and
- Research funding comes from a variety of sources: the researcher's own resources, grants from universities, CHRC, pharmaceutical companies, the regional private and public sectors, and international agencies (less than 10% comes from governments).

To summarize, the Caribbean region lacks a research culture, as reflected in the low level of government support and funding. Researchers feel that they have inadequate time, facilities, and infrastructure support. The number of full-time posts for researchers in universities, institutions, and government is thought to be much too small. Research administration and management are ineffective. Only just more than half of the current research relates to the regional health priorities. With some notable exceptions, the research to date has been primarily descriptive, epidemiological, and clinical. The research community communicates inadequately with the users of research (planners, policymakers, and the public in general). A wider range of stakeholders should be included in the research process; it should include, for example, the private sector, NGOs, trade and credit unions, religious groups, and the media. Including these groups as partners would facilitate the use of research.

IMPACT OF REGIONAL ORGANIZATIONS ON NATIONAL HEALTH RESEARCH

The following are some of the positive and negative impacts of regional organizations on health research in the region:

Positive impacts

- Researchers have a forum (annual scientific meeting) in which to present their work and get feedback from their peers and the network;
- A research-grant scheme assists young researchers beginning their careers;
- Training workshops in research skills and technology are available at both basic and advanced levels;
- Organizations convene workshops on common health problems, and this has resulted in the publication of clinical guidelines to manage conditions such as asthma, diabetes mellitus, and hypertension;
- Linkages and partnerships with researchers in other countries and donors are facilitated;
- Advocacy for health research occurs at the national level; and
- Advice is available on all aspects of research.

Negative aspects

- Some people have perceived CHRC as promoting esoteric research;
- Some have felt that CHRC competes with national groups for research funds;
- A number of researchers have become antagonistic because their papers were not accepted for the annual scientific meeting; and
- Some Health Ministry officials feel that they are too overburdened to help develop regional health-research initiatives.

REGIONAL HEALTH-RESEARCH PRIORITIES

Much attention has rightly gone to defining priority health areas. Yet, few Caribbean countries have defined national health-research priorities or a national health-research agenda. Although CCH II did not include a regional health-research agenda to match the eight health priorities, chief medical officers in the Caribbean have considered the creation of such an agenda a top priority for the region. In fact, the Caribbean has embarked on a process to identify its health-research agenda for the next decade, based on the eight health priorities. A Caribbean consultative process is under way.

There is a growing trend in the Caribbean to develop partnerships within and outside the region, and these partnerships are expected be one of the mechanisms to tackle these major health-research priorities.

THE WAY AHEAD

More countries in the Caribbean region need to establish ENHR and use this mechanism to define national priorities for health research. CHRC should strengthen its capability to promote and support ENHR in more countries and continue its program of training in research skills and methodology. The region should mobilize more resources to plan and implement priority health-research projects and programs. With the definition of regional health-research priorities currently under way, the Caribbean will have the opportunity to renew efforts to ensure that health research contributes strongly to the health of the people in the region.

CENTRAL AND EASTERN EUROPEAN COUNTRIES AND NEWLY INDEPENDENT STATES

Health-related research has a strong tradition in CEEC–NIS. Almost all the countries in the region once had or still have prominent scientific institutions and world-renowned scientists contributing to developments in their fields. From World War II until the end of the one-party regimes and planned economic systems, health research in Eastern European countries and the Soviet Union kept pace with global scientific progress, particularly in some areas of biomedicine and clinical research.

The health-related social sciences were in a considerably different position. For a long period, the behavioural sciences were a marginalized branch of health research. Furthermore, as a result of the political-economic system and its consequences for health care, some areas of research on health systems and health economics were either underdeveloped or missing entirely.

The socioeconomic changes at the end of the 1980s and the beginning of 1990s brought new challenges to health research. Most of the region's countries voted for a pluralistic, multiparty political system, and they all started to build the conditions for a market economy. This transition took place over a remarkably short period in the last decade. At the beginning of this transition, a deep economic crisis led to a considerable drop in the gross domestic products of these countries, and their financial capacities decreased. This led countries throughout the region to impose large-scale restrictive monetary measures, which obviously affected research financing as well. It became impossible to maintain the previous research capacities.

This was also a time of rapid social change and restructuring of societies, with mass unemployment, rising poverty, and changing societal norms and patterns. These trends resulted in new health risks. Life expectancy decreased in many countries — in some countries, such as the Russian Federation, the decrease in life expectancy was dramatic. The reform of health systems, including new methods of health-care financing, raised new questions for health-systems researchers.

To summarize, the socioeconomic transition of the past decade dramatically reduced funds for health research and posed new challenges for researchers in the fields of health-related behavioural sciences and health-systems research.

THE TRENDS OF THE PAST DECADE

Over the past 10 years, the state of health research in CEEC–NIS has reflected the overall socioeconomic crisis in the region. Countries attempted to maintain their research capacities under conditions of economic crisis and unbalanced state budgets. Nevertheless, most of the existing national health-research structures remained intact, together with financing mechanisms and career systems. The price of chronic underfunding, however, was a weakened research infrastructure and underpaid research staff. The consequence was a brain drain to the West and loss of a younger generation of researchers.

Globalization, increased involvement and research leadership of other countries, and rapid technical developments all helped to even further marginalize many of the region's research institutions or teams at a time when health-research systems were wrestling with financial difficulties. Some institutions managed to cope with these challenges, but in general the region's research centres lost their importance in terms of their contribution to global research.

Previous regional structures disintegrated; for example, cooperation dissolved between institutes within the framework of the Council of Mutual Economical Assistance and related bilateral and multilateral agreements. This happened in parallel with weakened or discontinued relationships in commerce, industry, and culture. The collapse of the Soviet Union and the rise of the independent republics have led to the disintegration of academic networks in the former Soviet republics as well.

Concurrently, researchers concentrated on establishing relationships with their counterparts in industrialized countries. This trend varied from country to country. It was most evident in the countries aiming to join the European Union (Central European, Baltic, and some Eastern European states). This reorientation of health research to new collaborative links and the simultaneous disintegration of regional structures led to a decline in the intensity of regional health-research cooperation.

THE PRESENT

Most health-research institutions successfully survived the first and probably the most difficult decade of the socioeconomic transition. The key to this was the strong and competitive pool of human resources and other nonmaterial resources: research traditions, scientific institutions, and the academic-scientific career system.

Health research is concentrated at state-run universities and academic institutions. The role of private-sector and nonprofit organizations is negligible except in countries that privatized their pharmaceutical industry, a move that resulted in some pharmaceutical research.

A competitive, merit-based resource-allocation system is in place in most countries, regardless of the subregion. Although most have set health-research priorities, funding does not always follow declared priorities; sometimes these priorities capture only a small portion of the available funds. Furthermore, the relevance of declared priorities to the actual health problems of the population is questionable, along with the quality of the priority-setting process. Weaknesses in the priority-setting process are partly attributable to the previous, antidemocratic regimes (including the communist and the preceding autocratic, antidemocratic regimes in most of CEEC–NIS). These traditions explain the lack of broad stakeholder and community involvement in priority-setting and the low emphasis on research concerning the sociocultural determinants of health (for example, inequality, ethnic minorities).

Another weak area is the poor research management found throughout the region — that is, the ineffectiveness of resource allocation and the inability to use available resources efficiently. The previous planned economies had no tradition of research management; they gave complete control of resource flows to their bureaucratic administrations. Thus, weak national and local research management accompanied the sharp decline in available funding, and this situation has persisted throughout the past 10 years.

EXISTING REGIONAL STRUCTURES

International partnerships within CEEC–NIS mostly take the form of bilateral cooperation involving individual researchers and institutions. These are thematic partnerships that focus on narrow fields of health research and use the structure of professional organizations. Although universities and academic institutions enter into some partnerships, most are personally initiated, involving joint projects and workshops.

One sees some good examples of subregional cooperation. These are often initiated by international organizations. In other cases, the scope of collaboration goes beyond the boundaries of the region. An excellent example is the Finland Baltic Health Monitoring of Adults program, which reflects cooperation between the Scandinavian and Baltic countries (Estonia, Latvia, and Lithuania). Initially, this was a collaboration of Finnish and Lithuanian partners; later, the other two Baltic republics joined. In addition, all of the Baltic states have good relations with the scientific organizations of the Scandinavian states, involving regular contacts between universities and research teams, mainly in the field of public health. WHO's Regional Office for Europe initiated CARIN. This network exchanges information on research subjects, projects, and results between the five former Soviet republics of Central Asia.

In the preaccession phase of the European Union, research institutes of Central European countries are eligible to participate in its research-project financing schemes. Depending on their country's agreement with the European Union, they can compete for research funds in cooperation with European partner institutes. Favouring this type of cooperation indicates the intention of the research communities of these countries to reorient their international partnerships, even if the socioeconomic conditions in Central European states differ remarkably from those of the European Union.

Overall, however, the region is far from fully exploiting its opportunities for partnerships in science and research, and the current relationships are only a fraction of those that were in place a decade ago.

LOOKING AHEAD

Regional cooperation would add great value to health research in CEEC–NIS. The basis of regional partnership might be a network of professional societies from various disciplines. The most appropriate approach to regional cooperation would be to follow the structure of subregions (for example, Central Europe, Eastern Europe and Russia, Central Asia). An important first step would be to establish a regional clearinghouse for research projects and results.

Furthermore, in the opinion of several health-research experts, CEEC–NIS definitely needs region-wide health-research training in local centres of excellence — this can serve as the basis for new institutions. A crucial issue with respect to regional cooperation would be the sustainability of these institutions, as the most common reason for terminating collaborative initiatives is lack of appropriate funding.

International organizations, such as WHO and COHRED, can contribute to building these structures by providing the basic expertise and methodology for effective networking, partnership development, and other aspects of strengthening national and regional health-research systems.

EASTERN MEDITERRANEAN

WHO's Regional Office for the Eastern Mediterranean has 23 countries under its purview, and they display a remarkable cultural, political, and socioeconomic diversity. Old civilizations with strongly entrenched cultural patterns are characteristic of the region, making systemic social change difficult and slow. Several countries have also suffered prolonged internal conflict. National populations range from just more than 600 000 in Bahrain to 139 million in Pakistan. More than 90% of the region's people live in low- to middle-income countries.

Despite the underfunding of health systems in many countries of the region, access to local health services and immunization coverage have improved. The profile of health conditions reflects the economic situation, with a high prevalence of vaccine-preventable and other communicable diseases in the poorest countries. Most new cases of tuberculosis have appeared in nine countries. Six countries have a severe malaria problem. The AIDS epidemic is spreading, although slowly, and the incidence of noncommunicable illnesses (including intentional and unintentional injuries) is rapidly increasing.

HEALTH-RESEARCH SITUATION

The wide diversity of the region's countries also appears in its profile of health research. Most countries now consider research an essential function of the health system, but they seldom apply research in formulating or revising health policies and programs. Demand for research from health planners and managers is minimal. Researchers and academicians are the ones who set research priorities, usually through consultations and workshops; in a few instances, they have used the results of health surveys. Countries in the region have made no attempt to broaden the base of stakeholders or establish some sort of national forum to discuss health-research issues. Coordination of health research within countries is weak and inefficient, having neither appropriate systems for research management nor transparent mechanisms to review and follow up on research proposals.

Few countries in the region have well-established research cultures to integrate research training into university education. Weaknesses appear at all stages of the research process: defining problems, data collection and analysis, and dissemination of results, including writing reports. With the exception of some short-term training courses and workshops, countries in the region have made no systematic or sustained efforts to strengthen the research capacities of their various stakeholders. This weak base also shows in the inability of researchers to tap external sources of funding and participate vigorously in regional and global debates on the future of health research.

REGIONAL STRUCTURES

The countries of this region are members of various political and economic forums, such as the Gulf Cooperation Council, the League of Arab States, Arab Ministers of Health, the Organization of Islamic States, and the Economic Cooperation Organization. However, they have no forum or regional structure for health research, other than those activities that the WHO regional office established and funds. The region has few functional health-research networks and, as a result, little intercountry collaborative research.

In 1976, WHO's regional office established its Advisory Committee on Health Research (ACHR), along with a system to award grants for research and research training. Since the early 1980s the directors of medical-research organizations or similar groups have met occasionally to exchange information and promote research on priority issues. WHO's regional office has supported, through its intercountry and national budgets, various national training activities in research methodology, management, and writing.

In 1986, stimulated by the global ACHR's proposed health-research strategy, the Eastern Mediterranean's ACHR created a regional task force to help countries establish national health-research policies and strategies. This task force visited 11 countries over a period of 9 years. As a result of this initiative, senior health managers learned about WHO's health-research policies and programs. The site visits also brought together researchers and health managers to discuss national health-research needs.

To strengthen national capacities for field-oriented research on prevalent tropical diseases, WHO's Regional Office for the Eastern Mediterranean and TDR jointly launched a small grants initiative in 1992. To date, it has invited seven rounds of applications; it has funded 78 of the 353 proposals received. Investigators in some countries have also benefited from technical and financial support from WHO special programs for research and training in human reproduction and tropical diseases. COHRED has been involved in the initiatives of only a small number of countries in the region.

TAKING STOCK AND LOOKING FORWARD

In June 2000, the region held a consultation to help prepare for the international conference in Bangkok. Representatives from 10 countries participated in this event, along with officials from the WHO regional office and some external observers. The participants identified strategic directions for health research for the coming decade and put forward specific recommendations, directing some to countries and others to regional and global support organizations.

A strong consensus emerged on several strategic directions. Examples include the importance of multistakeholder health-research forums and research priority-setting at not only national but also subnational and district levels. Participants urged WHO to take a more active and dynamic role in advocating the use of health research in health development and in the reduction of inequities in health. The participants recommended that the regional office serve as a prime mover to establish a regional health-research forum; they also recognized that ongoing leadership for health research in the region may need to come from other partners. The functions of the regional forum would include networking (for example, bridging arrangements between countries in the region and others in the North); identifying common regional problems, together with coordinating a regional research response to these problems; and serving as a platform to convey national concerns in various global research forums.

LATIN AMERICA[4]

In the 1990s, Latin America focused its attention on recovering from the financial crisis of the previous decade. This recovery appears in the S&T profiles of many Latin America countries:

— Investments in R&D increased substantially, by 57% between 1990 and 1996. Of this amount, more than 80% was in a small number of countries, notably Argentina, Brazil, Chile, and Mexico. Governments made more than 70% of these investments, and universities were the main recipients. Per capita investments in R&D in Argentina and Chile were 33.6 and 31.4 USD, respectively, compared with 25.0 USD for Brazil and 9.7 USD for Mexico (CONICYT 1998).

— The number of full-time equivalent researchers in Latin America rose to 125 000. Two countries accounted for more than two-thirds of this number: Brazil (50 000) and Argentina (28 500). The region had 0.75 researchers per 1 000 persons (in comparison with 3.25 in Spain, 5.51 in Canada, and 7.37 in the United States).

— In 1996, the publications of Latin American scientists represented 2.09% of all publications registered at the Institute for Scientific Information, compared with 1% in the 1970s and 1.5% in the 1980s. More than 60% of these publications were the work of scientists from Argentina, Brazil, Chile, and Mexico. The number of publications per 100 000 inhabitants for 1997 was 10.5 in Mexico and Chile, 9.5 in Argentina, and 3.5 in Brazil (CONICYT 1998).

---

[4] This section is adapted from a PAHO technical paper, "Science for Health," by Alberto Pellegrini Filho, Program Coordinator, Research Coordination Program, Division of Health and Human Development, PAHO, Washington, DC, USA.

The general health situation of Latin America has two prevailing characteristics. First, the region is rapidly going through demographic and epidemiological transitions, with declining fertility rates, decreasing mortality rates, and an aging population. It also shows striking health inequities, as seen in morbidity and mortality profiles and in access to health care. Some of this inequity is a consequence of the fragmentation of health services, which disadvantages the poor. Poor people spend nearly 6% of their household income on health care (compared with an average of 2.4% for all developing countries); in Colombia this figure is 12% and in Ecuador it is 17%.

The Latin American health-research community has in various ways attempted to respond to this situation. For example, recognizing the multiple determinants of health status, it has recently proposed a new paradigm of health research, with the following features:

— *Transdisciplinarity* — establishing links across disciplines while addressing important research problems;

— *Complexity* — ensuring that health research embraces broad conceptual models and avoids overly simplistic abstractions;

— *Multiplicity* — rejecting "monolithic" thought and looking for new and creative ways to address important problems; and

— *Praxis* — translating research findings into evidence-based clinical and public-health practice and into policies that feature high-impact interventions.

The capacity of the health-research community in Latin America to respond to these challenges has been analyzed. The numbers and distribution of health scientists correspond to the profile of S&T R&D. Only 2.7% of the publications of Latin American scientists deal with public-health issues. An analysis of all articles published by Latin American epidemiologists (60% of which were Brazilian) revealed that 83% dealt with infectious diseases, 4% with chronic noncommunicable illnesses, and 13% with other topics. This profile reflects a pretransitional pattern, not the pattern of currently prevailing conditions in the region.

Several initiatives are under way to reorganize health research for development. These include health-research priority-setting, financing, and dissemination and use of research results.

The issue of priority-setting was highlighted in an important 1998 publication, *Priorities in Collective Health Research in Latin America* (GEOPS 1998). A team of experts prepared a series of papers using "prospective analysis." This effort was promoted by the International Development Research Centre, PAHO, and COHRED. The Uruguay-based Study Group on Economics, Organization and Social Policies coordinated the entire initiative. This effort resulted in an important set of guidelines for determining the current and future agenda for public-health research in Latin America.

A trend in financial support in Latin America is increased funding, particularly from development banks and the private sector. Large international drug companies, for example, have supported clinical trials of new drug interventions. However, people have ethical concerns about using vulnerable groups for experimental populations — these groups are at some risk because they will in the long run be unable to afford the drugs. The World Bank and the Inter-American Development Bank are financing several projects in health-sector reform in many countries of the region, and each loan includes funding for operational studies. An assessment is necessary of the impact of these increased funds, particularly in regard to the use of research results and development of sustainable research capacity, and the system for judging the quality of research proposals should be stronger. *Quality* should include relevance and importance, along with scientific merit. The broader definition of *quality* would require both peer review (for scientific merit) and additional reviews involving representatives of stakeholder groups other than the researchers, such as decision-makers and other users of research.

For some time a large gap has existed between the production of knowledge and its dissemination and use. To strengthen the dissemination process, PAHO's Latin American and Caribbean Centre of Information in Health Sciences created a database of Latin American health-science literature. In addition, several Latin American health journals are now electronically accessible. PAHO has created a Virtual Health Library (VHL) on the Internet. Because a variety of users can access this service, it effectively reduces inequities in access to useful health information. Also under review are ways to provide scientific information to various groups of decision-makers, as each requires a unique type of evidence and poses a unique set of challenges in the dissemination and use of information.

THE STRUCTURE OF HEALTH RESEARCH

In most Latin American countries, the main national research institution is each country's Comisión Nacional de Investigación Cientifica y Tecnológica (CONICYT, national council for scientific and technological research). The United Nations Educational, Scientific and Cultural Organization and the Organization of American States helped to create these councils in the 1960s and 1970s. During the 1980s, many countries established research units within their ministries of health, often with PAHO's support. These units functioned as focal points within the CONICYT system. However, for the most part, they remain quite weak and have little influence on national research policies.

The institutions that actually conduct most health research are the universities and public organizations for S&T in health. In part as a consequence of less centralized planning, these institutions have recently become more visible, appearing as privileged actors with an opportunity to participate in defining S&T policies and plans. They have a dual challenge: to remain up to date on new advances in S&T and to respond effectively and efficiently to the problems of national societies and thereby maintain their social legitimacy.

PAHO INITIATIVES TO SUPPORT RESEARCH IN DEVELOPING COUNTRIES IN THE REGION

Through its research-grants program, PAHO has attempted to respond to the health-research needs of low-income countries in the region. Its basic strategy has been to promote networks and partnerships between research institutions on specific themes and projects. Some examples of projects are the following:

- Inequities in health status, access, and expenditure: using secondary data to inform policy-making (participating countries are Bolivia, Brazil, Colombia, Nicaragua, and Peru);

- A research competition on the theme of gender and equity in access to health care in reforms to health and social-security systems (projects were approved in six countries: Barbados, Brazil, Colombia, Chile, Ecuador, and Peru);

- A grant to the CONICYTs of Costa Rica and Guatemala to strengthen their development of public-health research; and

- A grant to the Latin American Biological Network to support research on infectious diseases and promote collaboration between laboratories with lower and higher levels of scientific infrastructure.

LESSONS ON THE ROLE OF REGIONAL ARRANGEMENTS IN STRENGTHENING NATIONAL RESEARCH

The following are some observations, based mostly on PAHO's experience, on the role of regional mechanisms to support and strengthen national systems to do equity-oriented health research for development:

— The creation of networks of research institutions has been an effective strategy for sharing resources and decreasing research-capacity gaps across countries. These networks have developed in the context of specific collaborative research projects and training programs, some of them explicitly focused on health inequities.

— Support to develop criteria, standards, and mechanisms for more cost-effective use of resources has led to the adoption of national systems (both peer and nonpeer review) to assess research proposals, using criteria of scientific merit, pertinence, relevance, and ethical compliance. The pattern of research-council funding is slowly changing, from an emphasis on research projects of interest only to researchers (mainly biomedical and clinical) to one that includes research to meet the needs of policymakers. A remaining practical challenge in most countries is to integrate a broader range of criteria (including policy relevance) into procedures for actually selecting projects.

— By explicitly promoting research policies that take account of the local context and feature problem-solving, countries in the region have been able to bring together both the producers and the users of research at all stages of the research process, from problem identification to the implementation and dissemination of results.

— The new ICTs constitute a good platform to support decentralized, participatory, problem-oriented research policies and programs (PAHO's VHL is an example of this).

CONCLUSIONS

Given the focus of this book, on national health-research systems, what observations can be made on these six regional perspectives? How have regional organizations and networks contributed to national efforts? What opportunities present themselves for future consideration? The following are the three general conclusions of this chapter:

— *Responsiveness to country needs* — Countries show a striking degree of diversity, even within a single region or subregion. We need to be reminded that Sierra Leone and Mauritius are in the same region — so are Bangladesh and Singapore; and Argentina and Haiti. These very different countries will have vastly different expectations of regional organizations. Thus, the message of country specificity, which pervades this book, applies as well to the role of regional organizations. Put another way, the needs of the member countries must drive the agendas of regional organizations (assuming their purpose is to serve the needs participating countries).

— *The added-value role of regional organizations* — Given the principle that regional entities should not be doing what countries can do, what then is the distinctive contribution of regional organizations and networks to health research for development? Again, the descriptions of the various regional structures are instructive, as they demonstrate a wide variety of goals. The more successful and sustained regional networks and organizations are those that meet specific needs and adapt to changing circumstances. For example, health researchers in the Caribbean live on islands with small populations; their need is for efficiency — a single agency (in this case, CHRC) provides links and services that it would be unrealistic to expect from individual island-states. Almost all the regional organizations described have mandates to facilitate information exchange among countries, improve efficiency through shared resources and expertise, provide technical and financial support, and advocate the needs of countries in the region at global forums.

— *Regional health-research forums* — Several regions have called for a regional health-research forum (notably Africa and the Eastern Mediterranean). In fact, the Caribbean has had such an intercountry forum for many years. As described above, regional health-research leaders in Asia recently created the Asian Forum for Health Research to serve as an informal consortium of country teams and regional organizations.

In addition to fulfilling some of the duties described above, a regional health-research forum can serve two other proactive functions. First, it can facilitate the creation of health-research and action coalitions to work on region-specific problems, particularly problems requiring an intersectoral response. Examples of such problems are the health risks of human migration and the impact of the drug and arms trade on human health. Second, a regional health-research forum can serve as an entry point for dialogue on the impacts of global trends on national health and social systems. The concerns of countries regarding globalization might then be more easily heard at a regional level, at least initially. An example of such an issue is the so-called jurisdiction gap, the phenomenon of there being more actors at the global level (notably transnational corporations) now than a decade ago, along with the real or merely perceived erosion of national sovereignty. Another example is the impact of structural-adjustment programs on health and education in the late 1980s and early 1990s, particularly in Africa. Research on this issue has received significant attention, in part because of regional intercountry collaboration.

Part III

THE WAY AHEAD

CHAPTER 8

COHRED AND ENHR: AN UPDATE AND LOOK AHEAD

Yvo Nuyens, Charas Suwanwela, and Nancy Johnson

SUMMARY

It is now 10 years after the Commission on Health Research for Development released its 1990 report. Essential National Health Research (ENHR) remains a vibrant strategy for achieving greater equity in health and a more integral role for research in development. Taken up in only a few countries in 1993, it has spread around the globe to nearly 60 countries.

In mid-1996, the Board of the Council on Health Research for Development (COHRED) commissioned an interim assessment of the ENHR strategy and of COHRED's performance in facilitating ENHR (COHRED 1996). The report of the external evaluation team drew attention to the need to capture and share country experiences on a set of "ENHR competencies" or "ENHR technology." The team also recommended more work on identifying indicators of ENHR success and a more comprehensive approach to capacity development that would include all stakeholders in the process. The COHRED Board responded by creating several task forces and working groups, involving members of the COHRED Board, national and regional research leaders, and other colleagues. Their tasks were to identify the requisite knowledge and skills for each competency, develop tool kits to assist ENHR planners in various countries, and address the capacity-development needs of national ENHR groups.

A 1999 internal review led to a sharpened sense of COHRED's institutional identity. COHRED stated its aims in three key messages: put countries first; work for equity in health; and link research to policy and action. One of COHRED's primary functions now is taking these messages to the countries and the international health research and development (R&D) community.

COHRED continues to provide technical support to countries engaged in ENHR, working with national research leaders to promote development-oriented health research, to set research priorities, to strengthen research mechanisms, and to build the capacities to do research and to use its results. It facilitates the interaction of leaders in health research, within and between countries. Countries share their experiences of creating a research environment to improve health and increase equity. Through printed and electronic publications, forums for discussion, and joint initiatives, COHRED facilitates experience-sharing among researchers, health workers, ministries of health, community organizations, and others. COHRED's regional- and country-level initiatives thus aim for the widest possible sharing of ideas and information.

Alongside preparations for the October 2000 international conference, past and present Board members reviewed COHRED's activities and possible future contribution. COHRED has an expanded role in supporting ENHR. It has a new set of messages and a stronger communication strategy.

To help countries improve their ENHR competencies, COHRED has provided tool kits, forums, and leadership training and has thereby established itself as a learning community, offering mutual encouragement and support among colleagues. It has developed partnerships with other health-research organizations, such as the World Health Organization (WHO) (headquarters and regional offices), the International Clinical Epidemiology Network (INCLEN), the Global Forum for Health Research (GFHR), and the Alliance for Health Policy and Systems Research, and it has helped to create networks and link countries with donors. COHRED now wants to strengthen these efforts and fashion coalitions with the widest range of stakeholders.

COHRED recently interviewed national research leaders and found that, in their view, ENHR should make simultaneous changes at all levels but keep its country focus. These national leaders gave four general recommendations, each discussed in detail in this chapter: local solutions for local problems, strengthened national leadership, greater regional cooperation, and a new deal with donors.

ENHR IN 2000

ENHR has caught on in Africa like wildfire because it's the kind of song we've been waiting for, for a long time. We want equity, we want consensus, we want to prioritize so that the little resources we have can be shared,

and we want to work together and network together. ENHR is the kind of philosophy we've been waiting for.
— Dr Mohamed Said Abdullah, National Health
Research and Development Centre, Kenya

Ten years after the Commission's 1990 report, ENHR remains a relevant and vibrant strategy for ensuring that countries derive real benefit from investments in health research. It works to acheive greater equity in health and to make research an active and integral part of development. From just a handful of countries in 1993, ENHR has spread around the globe. With COHRED acting as a facilitating mechanism, nearly 60 countries are currently implementing the ENHR strategy (see Box 8.1). Some of these countries are still in the exploratory start-up stage, whereas many others are well on the way to putting ENHR into practice. What is more, a number of other countries, programs, and networks have applied some of the underlying principles of ENHR without identifying themselves explicitly with the strategy (for example, the International Health Policy Program [IHPP], the Social Science and Medicine Africa Network, and Health Systems Research). Countries in five regions — Africa, Asia, the Caribbean, Eastern Europe–Central Asia, and Latin America — have pooled available technical and human resources to create a networking process for ENHR at the regional and, in some cases, at the subregional level (for example, the subregional ENHR network of French-speaking African countries).

Still, ENHR and COHRED have experienced inevitable growing pains. There are tales of success, as well as of failure, along the way. The preceding chapters have recounted many of the lessons learned. This chapter picks up the story of COHRED from where it left off in Chapter 1. It looks back at the role COHRED has played in support of ENHR, and it gives the views of COHRED's colleagues — national research leaders, in particular — on current challenges and the way ahead for COHRED and ENHR.

COHRED'S ROLE IN SUPPORT OF ENHR: ASSESSMENTS OF PAST PERFORMANCE

THE 1996 INTERIM ASSESSMENT

When COHRED was established in 1993, its primary role was to advocate ENHR and provide technical assistance on the seven strategic elements of ENHR (TFHRD 1991): promotion and advocacy, the ENHR mechanism, priority-setting, capacity-building and capacity-strengthening,

> **Box 8.1**
>
> ### The global spread of ENHR
>
> Countries engaged in the ENHR process are the following:
>
> | Africa | Asia | Eastern Europe–Central Asia |
> |---|---|---|
> | Benin | Bangladesh | Hungary |
> | Burkina Faso | Cambodia | Kazakhstan |
> | Burundi | China | Kyrgyzstan |
> | Cameroon | India | Lithuania |
> | Côte d'Ivoire | Indonesia | Tajikistan |
> | Egypt | Iran | Turkmenistan |
> | Ethiopia | Lao PDR | Uzbekistan |
> | Ghana | Malaysia | |
> | Guinea | Myanmar | **Latin America** |
> | Kenya | Nepal | Argentina |
> | Malawi | Oman | Brazil |
> | Mali | Pakistan | Chile |
> | Mauritius | Philippines | Colombia |
> | Mozambique | Thailand | Cuba |
> | Nigeria | Viet Nam | Mexico |
> | Senegal | | Nicaragua |
> | Seychelles | **Caribbean** | Venezuela |
> | South Africa | Curaçao | |
> | Sudan | Barbados | |
> | Swaziland | Jamaica | |
> | Tanzania | Trinidad and Tobago | |
> | Uganda | | |
> | Zambia | | |
> | Zimbabwe | | |

networking, financing, and evaluation. Over the next several years, with technical and, in some cases, financial assistance from COHRED, a number of countries initiated or extended their activities related to one or more of these elements. By mid-1996, the COHRED Board decided it was important to review the ENHR experience, so it commissioned an interim assessment of the strategy and of the council's performance. A four-person external evaluation team reviewed many relevant documents and interviewed key informants, donors, organizations, and leaders of research networks. The team also conducted site visits in seven countries, and one member of the team attended regional ENHR networking meetings in Africa and Asia.

The assessment team's report, *The Next Step: An Interim Assessment of* ENHR *and* COHRED (COHRED 1996), was tabled at a COHRED Board meeting in October 1996. Among the major observations was a statement of the need for a tool kit, or set of methods, to promote and implement ENHR. When ENHR was first launched and the Task Force on Health Research for Development identified the strategy's seven key elements, the Task Force assumed that people would see the need for these elements and implement them on their own. Indeed, that is what happened, and country ENHR groups implemented the seven strategic elements with various degrees of success. The interim-assessment team, however, drew attention to the need to capture and share country experiences of ENHR competencies, and it recommended meeting this need "through the systematic application of a knowledge and skills base" (COHRED 1996, p. 29). These competencies (also referred to as "ENHR technology") included the original seven strategic elements, plus two new ones: community participation and the translation of research into policy and action (see Figure 8.1). The team went on to suggest that "the definition, elaboration and use of this technology represents COHRED's niche, its value added contribution to the global health and development endeavour" (COHRED 1996, p. 29).

Although COHRED had made some progress in defining indicators of ENHR success, it needed to do more work to move beyond process description to analysis of impacts and outputs. As well, the team noted that in many instances capacity-building focused primarily on researchers. It recommended a more comprehensive approach to capacity development for ENHR, to include all stakeholders: policymakers, communities, their NGO representatives, donors, the media,

Essential National Health Research

Goals
Put countries first
Work for equity
Link research to policy and action

Competencies
Promotion and advocacy
Building an innovative mechanism
Priority-setting
Capacity-strengthening
Research mobilization
Linking research to action and policy
Community participation
Network- and coalition-building
Evaluation

Figure 8.1. ENHR goals and competencies.

health professionals, and the private sector. (A summary of the recommendations made in the interim assessment report appears in Box 8.2.)

The COHRED Board vigorously debated these observations and suggestions and then quickly moved to implement their spirit and substance, creating several task forces and working groups. COHRED's Task Force on ENHR Competencies (comprising four working groups) was created to look at priority-setting; research to policy and action; promotion, advocacy, and the ENHR mechanism; and community participation. COHRED established two other task forces, one on resource flows and the other on evaluation and critical indicators of success. A year later, at its 1997 annual meeting, the Board created the Advisory Committee on Health Research Capacity Strengthening, thus recognizing that this issue pervades many aspects of the ENHR process.

The various groups — involving members of the COHRED Board, national and regional research leaders, and other colleagues — took responsibility for identifying the requisite knowledge and skills for each competency, developing tool kits to assist ENHR planners in various countries, and providing training for national ENHR groups. (Specific objectives of a number of COHRED working groups and task forces are listed in Box 8.3.) Although these groups are currently at diverse stages in their work, several have begun to produce a variety of materials, including manuals, evaluation tools, issues papers, pamphlets, and learning briefs (see Box 8.4) (available through the COHRED Secretariat). Others have been less successful. The Resource Flows Task Force failed to get off the ground; instead, COHRED undertook several intercountry studies, which it used to provide input into GFHR's Core Group on Resource Flows. COHRED's Critical Indicators Task Force developed a survey instrument to enable countries to assess their progress in ENHR. However, the evaluation tool proved too cumbersome, and the work of this task force has stalled.

THE 1999 INTERNAL REVIEW

In February 1999, an ad hoc group of COHRED associates joined the COHRED Coordinator and the Board Chair in Geneva to conduct an informal, internal review of COHRED's role and performance. They reflected on the "new realities" in the global community and the international health-research sector (see Chapter 9), as well as on the challenges these present for COHRED. Among these new realities are the growing importance of knowledge management and innovative use of communication technologies, the emergence of several new

Box 8.2

Recommendations of the interim assessment report

1. **Product: training in ENHR technology**
    - Create a special initiative to capture the available expertise regarding the competencies which comprise "ENHR technology," prepare strategies and materials ("tool kits"), and provide training to country ENHR groups. (COHRED 1996, p. 29).

2. **Partnerships: purpose-specific coalition-building**
    - Create regional "ENHR mentoring teams" to assist countries with coalition building, particularly in the early stages of the ENHR process where "political mapping" is most important. Where possible, these mentoring teams should include representatives of the three core partners — researchers, policymakers, and community groups; in some situations, a donor representative could be added (COHRED 1996, p. 31).
    - Establish a task force to explore specific ways in which national and global research initiatives can be linked. The task force should be initiated by COHRED, and include representatives of the WHO [World Health Organization] and other UN agencies, and the World Bank, aiming to develop exemplary collaborative projects and programs at the country level (COHRED 1996, p. 32).

3. **People: comprehensive research capacity-strengthening**
    - Broaden the scope of research training beyond the usual researcher community; COHRED should identify countries where there may already be experience with a broader scope of research training, with the aim of strengthening and disseminating this experience (COHRED 1996, p. 32).
    - Initiate one or more country case studies focused on this issue; these studies would be not only analytic and descriptive, but would proactively propose and implement solutions to ensure that potentially available research expertise is contributing to the ENHR process (COHRED 1996, p. 33).
    - Facilitate special initiatives with appropriate networks and institutions to introduce ENHR concepts and skills to the curricula that prepare future health professionals. This initiative should feature opportunities for students to participate directly in all aspects of the ENHR plan (COHRED 1996, p. 33).

4. **Performance: a stronger COHRED**
    - COHRED Board should become more "problem-oriented" in the way it functions. This could be achieved by forming small short term task force groups to deal with special relevant issues. Also, the COHRED Board could be more efficient either by creating a small executive committee where each member has a specific responsibility or by reducing its size (COHRED 1996, p. 34).
    - COHRED Secretariat should be strengthened to increase its capacity for specific analytic projects. This could be done either by adding a professional officer to the Geneva-based unit, or by engaging regionally based professionals on a part-time basis (COHRED 1996, p. 35).

Source: COHRED (1996, excerpts from pp. 29–35).

> **Box 8.3**
>
> ### COHRED task-force and working-group objectives
>
> **Task Force on ENHR Competencies (WG1–4)**
>
> **WG1 Priority Setting**
> — To review country experiences with priority-setting for ENHR
> — To develop a framework for ENHR priority-setting, focusing on an analysis of health needs, people's expectations, and societal trends and based on lessons learned from countries
> — To produce orientation and training materials on priority-setting for use by countries
>
> **WG2 Research to Action and Policy**
> — To identify key variables, links, and mechanisms in the transfer process of research into action and policy, by reviewing, analyzing, and synthesizing experiences from organizations, programs, institutions, and countries
> — To develop process–mechanisms for use by countries in improving the transfer from research to policy
>
> **WG3 Promotion, Advocacy and the ENHR Mechanism**
> — To document successful examples, facilitating and constraining factors, and generic and country-specific lessons in promoting and institutionalizing ENHR
> — To develop a range of learning instruments for improving knowledge and skills within countries and related strategies in promoting and institutionalizing ENHR
> — To evaluate the impact of learning instruments and strategies after their application within a series of countries
>
> **WG4 Community Participation**
> — To review the context, process, and outcomes of community participation in the ENHR strategy as practiced in a series of countries
> — To document examples of community involvement in order to show modalities worked out in various countries
> — To use the examples to discuss problems as well as best practices
> — To extract lessons learned
>
> **Resource Flows Task Force**
> — To review existing methodologies to estimate and monitor resource flows for health research
> — To voice concerns, experiences, and interests of developing countries in the global dialogue on this issue
> — To facilitate and support case studies in and by countries in this area
> — To strengthen capacities of countries in setting up a monitoring system on resource flows
>
> *(continued)*

Box 8.3 concluded.

Critical Indicators Task Force
— To construct a set of critical indicators to demonstrate the added value of the ENHR approach
— To facilitate countries and regions in assessing their progress in implementing the ENHR strategy
— To develop a monitoring system for COHRED and its constituents, stakeholders, and interested partners

Advisory Committee on Health Research Capacity Strengthening
— To develop and promote a comprehensive approach to health-research capacity development
— To sensitize partner organizations already involved in health-research capacity development to enable countries to independently assess their capacity-development–ENHR needs and implement a corresponding capacity-development strategy for health research
— To mobilize financial, human, and institutional resources for this capacity-development–ENHR initiative, which has a high potential to contribute to more equity in health status and health research

Box 8.4

Selected COHRED publications

Country monographs

1. Essential National Health Research in Uganda: a case study of progress and challenges in implementing the ENHR strategy. Prepared by the Uganda National Health Research Council. COHRED document 2000.6

2. ENHR in the Philippines: the first five years 1991–1996. Abaya, E. et al. 1997 COHRED document 97.5

3. ENHR development in Thailand. Chunharas, S.; Chooprapawan, C. 1997. COHRED document 97.6

4. ENHR in South Africa. Jeenah, S. et al. 1997. COHRED document 97.7

5. ENHR in Kenya. The National Health Research and Development Centre. 1998. COHRED document 98.2

6. Evolution of health research essential for development in Ghana. Adjei, S.; Gyapong, J. 1999. COHRED document 99.3

7. Essential National Health Research in Bangladesh, an ENHR country monograph. Hossain, M. 2000. COHRED document 2000.1

(continued)

Box 8.4 concluded.

Evaluation tools

8. ENHR — a strategy for action in health and human development. Task Force on Health Research for Development. 1991; pages 44–47 deal specifically with evaluation (also available in French)

9. How effective is your country's strategy for health research? Annex to Health research: powerful advocate for health and development, based on equity. COHRED Working Group on Promotion, Advocacy and the ENHR Mechanism. 2000. COHRED document 2000.2

Issues papers

10. How to boost the impact of country mechanisms to support ENHR. A peek into the melting pot of country experiences. COHRED Working Group on Promotion, Advocacy and the ENHR Mechanism. 1999. COHRED document 99.1 (French version: COHRED Document 99.2)

11. Health research: powerful advocate for health and development, based on equity; COHRED Working Group on Promotion, Advocacy and the COHRED Mechanism. 2000. COHRED document 2000.2

12. Community participation in essential national health research. S. Reynolds Whyte for the COHRED Working Group on Community Participation. 2000. COHRED document 2000.5

Manuals

13. A manual for research priority setting using the ENHR Strategy. Okello, D.; Chongtrakul, P. and the COHRED Working Group on Priority Setting. 2000. COHRED Document 2000.3

14. The ENHR handbook. A guide to Essential National Health Research. COHRED Document 2000.4

Regional reports

15. African Conference on Health Research for Development: conference programme and country reports, 19–23 September 1999, Zimbabwe

16. Proceedings 3rd Asian Regional Meeting on Essential National Health Research, 11–12 December 1998, Lao PDR

17. Report of the Fifth African ENHR Network Conference, 5–7 October 1998, Ghana

18. Proceedings ENHR Asia, 2nd Regional Meeting, 9–11 December 1997, Viet Nam

19. Summary report on the Workshop of the Central and East European Network on Essential National Health Research, 9–14 November 1997, Hungary

20. Regional workshop on Essential National Health Research and Priority Setting in Health Research, 6–8 November 1995, Jamaica

international health-research organizations, and the concern, of late, that equity has fallen off global and national health-research agendas in favour of efficiency-based health reforms.

An analysis of strengths, weakness, opportunities, and threats resulted in a sharpened sense of COHRED's institutional identity and how it complements the goals of the many other international health-research organizations and initiatives, such as WHO, GFHR, and the Scientists for Health Research and Development. COHRED captured its niche in three key messages:

— Put countries first;

— Work for equity in health; and

— Link research to policy and action.

These messages have become the core of the newly energized COHRED communication strategy, which harnesses the latest communication technologies. COHRED has subsequently devised an electronic library and a number of paper and electronic promotional materials, such as *The ENHR Handbook* (COHRED 2000c). The electronic library now enables the COHRED Secretariat to respond faster and more effectively to requests for specific or customized information. In the future, it will provide direct access to these materials through the COHRED website (http://www.cohred.ch) or a CD-ROM database.

COHRED'S KEY MESSAGES

A recent COHRED issue paper, "Health Research: Powerful Advocate for Health and Development Based on Equity" (COHRED 2000e), provides a full discussion of each of the key messages, including ways of reaching the objective contained in the message and the risks involved. The remainder of this section briefly describes each of these three messages (based on the issue paper).

PUT COUNTRIES FIRST

> *However poor a country may be, it should use its limited resources to ensure that it does the research that is relevant to its people.*
> — Professor Raphael Owor, Faculty of Medicine,
> Makerere University, Uganda

> *There are always problems which are unique to a country which need to be dealt with effectively and efficiently, and this cannot be achieved by borrowing a research agenda from another country.*
> — Dr Izzy Gerstenbluth, Department of Epidemiology and Research, Medical and Public Health Service of Curaçao, Curaçao

Perhaps the strongest argument for putting countries first is the tremendous success of those nations that have done exactly that. Self-interest has driven R&D in developed countries — such as Japan, the United States, and those in Western Europe — to great effect. Obviously, owing to limited resources, developing countries face a tremendous challenge in investing in R&D. However, the point remains that national research efforts that respond directly to specific health problems have had the most success.

Current trends in globalization and increasing inequities make the country focus even more important, particularly a focus on the poorest, most marginalized countries. Although technologies are now available to rapidly disseminate new knowledge around the world, the reality is that developed countries are the main beneficiaries — the "globalization of knowledge" is a misnomer. Privatization of research, tighter intellectual property rights, and the growing gap in access to communication technologies are all factors working against the interests of the poor in developing countries. Although these countries try to take advantage of the "global economy," they need to ensure that the concerns of their people are not lost in the process.

The objectives of national research in developing countries are at least fourfold. The first is to make more effective use of existing knowledge, technologies, and health interventions. In some cases, this may mean adapting knowledge and technologies for local use; in others, it will mean making current interventions more efficient and effective. A second objective is to make currently effective (yet expensive) interventions simpler and more affordable. Often, this will involve collaboration with researchers from other countries where people experience similar health problems. A third objective is to participate in research to discover new ways of dealing with priority problems. In some instances, developing countries may get involved in the research; in others, they may only advocate research to address their priorities, without necessarily participating in it. Their advocacy may focus on international investors and agencies, as well as on researchers in developed countries. A fourth objective is to protect against misinformation and exploitation; for example, manufacturers and distributors of pharmaceutical and health products in developing countries often use distorted information, together with incentives, when marketing their products. The tobacco industry has used similar tactics, such as misinforming people about filtered cigarettes.

WORK FOR EQUITY IN HEALTH

> *Health must be seen as an integral part of economic development. Then equitable distribution of health resources would become part of larger political movements.*
> — Dr Michael Phillips, Research Centre of Clinical Epidemiology, Beijing Hui Long Guan Hospital, China

> *Each country is responsible for putting equity up front.*
> — Dr Lye Munn Sann, Institute of Medical Research, Malaysia

Left to market forces and curiosity alone, health research would tend to reflect the priorities and health problems of the rich. Instead of helping to narrow the gap between rich and poor, it would simply widen existing disparities. Health research should actively work to eradicate such disparities. Underpinning this argument is the belief in the worth of every individual and the belief that every person is entitled to realize that worth.

Another compelling argument is that health for all promotes national development. Countries impede their economic growth and social development by underinvesting in the health of the poor. A high burden of disease — found largely among the poorest countries — hinders both economic growth and human development and limits international competitiveness. We now see evidence that equity-oriented strategies contribute directly to economic growth.

Working for equity also improves efficiency. Countries can make the biggest reduction in the burden of disease if they concentrate on improving the health status of those who carry the heaviest burden of disease, and these are almost invariably the poor and other marginalized groups.

Unlike improvements in the health status of wealthier nations, which will require dramatic technological breakthroughs to make giant leaps forward, relatively small investments in the application of existing knowledge can substantially improve the health of at least some of the poor. Efforts to further reduce the burden of disease through existing technologies depend largely on enhanced technical efficiency, better allocation of resources, and greater cost-effectiveness.

With local knowledge and customized application, we can squeeze far more benefit out of new or existing interventions. In many African countries, for example, people widely access both the traditional and the Western health-care systems. A growing concern has been that some practices of African traditional healers place them and their patients at risk for HIV–AIDS. Healers may use the same razor to scarify several patients, take a patient's blood into their own mouth in the practice of "biting out," or rub herbal medicines into open cuts with unwashed hands. Ethnographic research has highlighted the importance of the sociopolitical and cultural context of healing practices, as well as indigenous understanding of AIDS, in developing a culturally appropriate HIV–AIDS educational intervention in which traditional healers collaborate in identifying risky therapeutic practices and in finding and applying solutions (Willms et al. 1996).

LINK RESEARCH TO POLICY AND ACTION

> *In Indonesia research is still something that looks serious and something policymakers feel is not really important to do because they can decide by themselves. Another problem is also that the environment is not really supportive of research. Research is said to be expensive and so on.*
> — Dr Agus Suwandono, Health Services Research and Development Centre, National Institute of Health Research for Development, Ministry of Health, Indonesia

> *A key challenge is to make research demand-driven and to sensitize researchers to the needs and priorities that are in the national interest.*
> — Dr Lye Munn Sann, Institute of Medical Research, Malaysia

The private sector is driven by profit and zeal to yield the best rate of return on investment. Perhaps that is why the private rather than the public sector leads the way in redefining processes of innovation and replacing fairly static and step-by-step approaches with more dynamic and interactive ones. The priorities of private industry differ in many important ways from those of the public sector, especially the public sector's global role in safeguarding and promoting fundamental research. Nevertheless, researchers working to promote health can learn much from the experience of technological development.

Weak demand for research may lead to inefficient outcomes: the failure of research to meet the needs of potential users; or even the complete neglect of important research topics. This has several implications:

- Researchers in developing countries with severe resource shortages may handicap themselves even more if they do not make the most efficient use of these scarce resources (many developing-country researchers were trained in developed countries in programs emphasizing research design and methodology, rather than planning and management);

- Researchers and national research coordinators can engage with user groups to stimulate demand for research and thereby improve the efficiency of the research process; and

- Although there is demand for research to improve the health of the poor — at least by the poor — this demand is not revealed in the market for research. This leads to an underinvestment in pro-poor research.

Some concrete ways to overcome these inefficiencies would be to promote research by the poor themselves and to link research to action to improve the health of the poor. (See Chapter 4 on participatory research and empowerment.)

Linking research to action can improve the quality of research as well. Testing and revising knowledge by applying it to real-world problems can strengthen the quality of the research, rather than compromising it. This is an important argument to make with people in the academic community, who are less likely to be persuaded by the above-mentioned arguments of effectiveness or efficiency.

CURRENT ROLE AND ACTIVITIES

Currently, COHRED's primary function is to take its three messages to developing countries and the international health R&D community. COHRED also continues to provide technical support to countries implementing ENHR. It works with national research leaders to promote health research as a tool for development, establish research priorities, strengthen mechanisms to support research, and build research and user capacities. Specifically, it facilitates the interaction between health-research leaders, within and between countries. In this way, it helps these countries share experiences and insights into creating a stimulating research environment focused sharply on the goals of better health and greater equity. COHRED also provides an active forum for sharing experiences of ENHR. Through a series of printed and electronic publications, forums for discussion, and joint initiatives, COHRED is enabling researchers, health workers, ministries of health, community organizations, and others to share experiences and learn from one another. COHRED's regional- and country-level initiatives aim to share information and ideas as widely as possible.

REGIONAL NETWORKING ACTIVITIES

Africa

Just over a year after the creation of COHRED, the first African ENHR networking meeting convened in Mombassa, Kenya (May 1994). The participants (more than 30 individuals from seven African countries) recognized the value of sharing country experiences of ENHR and strongly recommended that such meetings be held regularly. As a result, the regional network has been holding these meeting each year in various African locations (Accra, Arusha, Harare, Kampala). Professor Raphael Owor of Uganda was the first regional network coordinator; he was succeeded in 1999 by Dr Steve Chandiwana of Zimbabwe. These meetings have been contiguous with others, such as the Fourth Africa ENHR meeting in Arusha, held in conjunction with a special conference on health policy in Africa (which IHPP cosponsored) and the World Conference of Public Health Associations. A joint meeting of ENHR, the African Clinical Epidemiology Network, and the Public Health School Without Walls took place in Kampala, in October 1996. A subregional network for French-speaking countries has operated for the past several years, providing a subregional francophone coordinator. The regional network has established communication links with other African regional health-research organizations, in part as an outcome of a "networking-the-networks" meeting held in January 1996, in conjunction with a global meeting of INCLEN held in Victoria Falls.

The African ENHR Mentoring Team manages the program and activities of the network. This team includes the regional coordinator and African members of the COHRED Board. It has taken on various functions, such as providing advice and support for individual countries, liaising with the COHRED Secretariat and Board and regional organizations (such as the WHO Regional Office for Africa), and planning the annual ENHR networking meeting. To prepare for the October 2000 conference in Bangkok, the Mentoring Team has participated in an intensive consultation process to ensure that a strong and clear "African voice" speaks for Africa at the conference.

Asia

Representatives have been meeting from Asian countries engaged in the ENHR strategy: their first meeting was in Thailand in 1995, followed by meetings in the Philippines (1996), Viet Nam (1997), and Lao PDR (1998). The Asian ENHR network has created collaborative regional task forces and project groups, such as working groups on resource flows and a regional study on equity. It rotates its secretariat every 2 years. Bangladesh initially hosted the network, followed by the Philippines and, currently, Thailand. Regional cooperation has characterized a number of national activities, such as priority-setting workshops in Indonesia, Lao PDR, Nepal, and Viet Nam and a training workshop on research management and networking, in Thailand.

During the past year, the Asian ENHR network has been involved in an intensive review of the status of health research for development in Asia in preparation for the Bangkok conference. It has attempted specifically to "widen the circle" and involve as many Asian groups with direct involvement in health research as possible. To do this, it made innovative use of information and communication technologies over the several months leading up to the dynamic Asian Forum on Health Research, in Manila in February 2000.

The Caribbean

The Commonwealth Caribbean Medical Research Council (CCMRC) (now the Caribbean Health Research Council [CHRC]) strongly facilitated the introduction and development of ENHR in the Caribbean region (specifically, the 18 English-speaking countries and the Netherlands Antilles). At the November 1995 joint CCMRC–COHRED workshop in Jamaica, teams from five countries discussed issues of priority-setting for health research, and they prepared country ENHR plans. Four of the five countries presented progress reports in April 1996 at a meeting of CCMRC in Trinidad.

As the regional ENHR networking body, CCMRC also created a dedicated position for an ENHR scientist. Between September 1995 and May 1998, this scientist supported processes for preparation and prioritization of research proposals and organized workshops on research skills.

During a regional consultation in 1997, the Caribbean Cooperation in Health (CCH) initiative identified eight health-research priorities for the region, along with strategies for implementation and joint action. CCMRC became CHRC and began the process of defining a regional health-research agenda for the eight priorities. So far, four countries in the region have established ENHR committees: Barbados, Curaçao, Jamaica, and Trinidad and Tobago.

Eastern Europe–Central Asia

Eastern Europe launched its network-building process through the leadership of Dr Peter Makara. In June 1996, a workshop was jointly organized by the Hungarian National Institute for Health Promotion, COHRED, and the International Forum for Social Sciences in Health. This was followed in November 1997 by the Workshop on Inequity and Health: From Research to Policies. Participants discussed building the capacity of Central and Eastern European countries and the Baltic states for research, policy, and action to meet the challenges of inequity in the region, which include poverty, social exclusion, unemployment, migration, homelessness, minority issues, and other important aspects of socioeconomic disadvantage.

In 1999, the Bishkek Declaration extended the regional network to include the Central Asian republics and Kazakhstan (CARK). A workshop was held with representatives from the CARK countries, researchers, and members of the CARK Mother and Child Health Forum. Many international agencies and donors attended the workshop, including COHRED, the WHO Regional Office for Europe, the United Nations Children's Fund, the United Nations Fund for Population Activities, the Centres for Disease Control, and the World Bank. Participants made a commitment to adopt ENHR.

Recently, the network also undertook a regional consultation to help develop its health-research agenda for the next decade and prepare for the conference in Bangkok.

Latin America

In November 1999, the Latin America region launched a consultation process to prepare for the Bangkok conference. Similar to consultations in the other regions, it involved representatives from a number of existing networks (the Latin American and Caribbean Women's Network, INCLEN, and the Health Systems and Services Research Network in the Southern Cone), various government agencies (Health ministries and science and technology councils), and a number of universities. It culminated in a synthesis meeting in Buenos Aires, in June 2000, where the various participants purposed forming a more permanent link (that is, a network of networks). The momentum created by the consultation process, it is hoped, will carry over, with participating countries strengthening their health-research systems through a clear orientation in favour of equity and social and gender justice.

FUTURE DIRECTIONS FOR COHRED

In parallel with the many preparations for the October 2000 conference, COHRED continued to review its activities of the last several years, as well as look ahead to its possible future contribution. Past and present COHRED Board members participated in this process, which has clarified the council's future tasks and roles.

COHRED has broadened its role in support of ENHR. It continues to serve as an advocate of ENHR, but with a newly articulated and focused set of messages, as well as a stronger communication strategy. When country groups asked for support to improve their ENHR competencies, COHRED responded with tool kits, forums for sharing country experiences, and leadership training. In doing so, it has become a learning community and a collegium in which colleagues encourage and support each other in the ongoing work of achieving COHRED's goals: putting countries first, working for equity in health, and linking research to action. As it looks ahead to the next decade, COHRED envisions an enhanced role as broker of coalitions and partnerships. Thus far, it has developed partnerships with like-minded organizations, such as WHO (headquarters and regional offices), INCLEN, GFHR, and the Alliance for Health Policy and Systems Research; worked to create networks; and helped to link countries with donors. COHRED would like to strengthen its efforts in these areas and build coalitions with the widest possible range of stakeholders.

The organization sees the following as its key tasks for the coming years as it fulfills each of the four roles described above:

As an advocate

— Sharpening its communication strategy;

— Changing the perception that ENHR is for poor countries only;

— Finding ways to get the "country voice" into international research;

— Emphasizing that ENHR is not another vertical program; and

— Correcting the perception that COHRED is a mobile bank.

As a broker

— Working with countries to see how coalitions can effect change;

- Building effective research networks among developing countries; and
- Acting as a broker with donors.

As a learning community
- Strengthening leadership for research management and promotion; and
- Identifying and preparing the next generation of leaders for COHRED.

As a collegium
- Continuing to foster the development of regional ENHR structures; and
- Building links with other global partners.

Additionally, COHRED will work to develop qualitative and quantitative measures of ENHR's success and COHRED's own performance. This will entail, among other things, choosing a definition of *equity* and making it practical by describing specific gauges and initiatives to promote and measure equity trends.

VIEWS OF NATIONAL RESEARCH LEADERS

Between July 1999 and May 2000, COHRED collected the views of a number of national research leaders on key challenges and future directions for ENHR. On an opportunistic basis, it invited 19 national research leaders to participate in in-depth interviews. All agreed to the interviews, and relevant portions of each were transcribed. A document analysis of the reports of four site visits conducted during the African consultation also offered some interesting perspectives.

The overarching message from national leaders was that ENHR must work to simultaneously effect change at the local (community and district), national, regional, and global levels, but without losing its focus on countries. Specifically, the research leaders called for the following:

- Local solutions for local problems;
- Strengthened national leadership;
- Greater regional cooperation; and
- A new deal with donors.

To let the voice of the national research leaders come through, the remainder of this chapter presents direct quotations from these individuals and from the reports of the site visits, followed by a short summary of the key points that the participants raised under each of the above recommendations. (Appendix 8.1 provides a list of these individuals and of the site-visit reports used.)

LOCAL SOLUTIONS FOR LOCAL PROBLEMS

The real business is at the district level. Needed are researchers who are oriented to the community and have experience conducting district level research.... Research at the community and district level is able to identify where inequities are and the means of correcting them can even be local.... The health research system has not yet penetrated local levels enough to help identify inequities and correct them. I think we are still at the national top level and we need to put research at a lower level in order to achieve that.
— Professor Raphael Owor, Faculty of Medicine, Makerere University, Uganda

A major challenge is to really work with all three stakeholders. So far, the community has been neglected. Researchers are not trained to perceive communities as real stakeholders. When we invite "the community," we invite NGOs but they are NOT the community. Communities are not professionals, therefore they need a different approach, based on partnership and understanding. If we really want to work with them, we need researchers who are engaged, and researchers who can dedicate enough time to understand the culture they work in.
— Benin site-visit report

The role of traditional healers in research is not clear, yet they are very important stakeholders. There is a need to value and elaborate on their possible contribution to ENHR and equity in development.
— Benin site-visit report

Health-research priority-setting should follow a bottom-up rather than top-down approach. Local (community and district) health problems and needs should drive national health-research agendas, and the resulting policies and programs must be locally appropriate, taking account of the social, cultural, economic, and political context. Community members need to have a real voice in determining health-research priorities, and the researchers should empower them to find solutions to their health problems. Traditional healers, along with women's groups and other previously overlooked segments of the community, should be counted among the various stakeholder groups and given equal respect. The local level is where we are likely to realize the greatest improvements in equity.

STRENGTHENED NATIONAL LEADERSHIP

A comprehensive approach to strengthening national leadership must go beyond skills training and recognize the fundamental need to change attitudes, values, and motivations in research, health, and equity. Without such changes, we are unlikely to achieve a pro-equity political agenda, allocate greater resources to health research, link research to action, or build research capacity.

Achieving a pro-equity political agenda

> *Politicians prefer solving the kinds of problems that can be addressed over the short term rather than the long term. They have a four-year term in which to make some perceptible difference in the eyes of the general voting population. What can they achieve in that time? It's pretty rare that you will find a politician who is willing to transcend his own political career — to look past the 4-year term and see that putting money into health research will make a difference in the long term.*
> — Dr Izzy Gerstenbluth, Department of Epidemiology and Research, Medical and Public Health Service of Curaçao, Curaçao

Research has helped greatly to elucidate inequities. Doing something about them also requires political will. Research may help to formulate and evaluate policy options, but a pro-equity political agenda is paramount. Much political will (and, consequently, research) focuses on improving the efficiency of health systems. It is assumed that greater efficiency will create savings, which can in turn be redistributed to the benefit of the poor; in addition, decision-makers like to focus on problems for which they can find a "quick fix."

Allocating greater resources to health research

> *African countries must put research higher on the agenda and give money for real research, not just money to maintain vehicles for the directors of the institute, or to maintain buildings; that is not enough. We need money to be put into the research process itself.... Funding for health research must be built into national budgets — even if budgets are supported largely by international agencies rather than local taxes.... What I have been trying to tell them is, "Look, if you can beg to build a health centre why don't you beg also for health research?" I think this has sunk in. The strategic plan*

of the Ministry of Health this year is such that it includes research — which it has never done before.
— Professor Raphael Owor, Faculty of Medicine, Makerere University, Uganda

No matter how poor the country, national leadership must make research a priority and allocate a portion of its budget accordingly.

Linking research to action

We were always concerned that policy was only ever developed on an ad-hoc basis, and more often than not, it was financially geared. So, we decided to try and change this trend. We wanted policy to be based on research, hard facts, or real information.
— Dr Izzy Gerstenbluth, Department of Epidemiology and Research, Medical and Public Health Service of Curaçao, Curaçao

A major challenge has been changing the mindset of the past generation of policymakers and convincing people of the vital role research plays in national development and trying to inculcate a research culture and institutionalizing that. A key strategy was to gain commitment at the highest level in recognizing and supporting research as an important factor in development.
— Dr Lye Munn Sann, Institute of Medical Research, Malaysia

Governments need to develop a culture of evidence-based, transparent, and accountable decision-making. To bridge research and policy, we also need research managers who can communicate with both sides and understand the policy uses and implications of research.

Strengthening research capacity

Unless we change our attitude toward our researchers and give them incentives, give them career structures, they will go away.
— Dr Akhtar Ali Qureshi, Health Services Academy, Ministry of Health, Pakistan

In Bénin the university is still in its infancy. Most of Bénin's researchers are trained abroad and don't come back. Researchers face competing demands on their time. The main causes of the brain drain are insufficient local incentives compared to foreign offers and unfavourable working conditions. Local capacity is being supplemented by external visiting researchers but the inflow is not significant. They mostly collaborate in the fields of community health, health-care financing, and clinical research. Contribution to capacity development is limited to providing equipment. Most of the foreign researchers work according to the priorities set by their (foreign) institution.
— Benin site-visit report

> *In the newspaper, I read an article on brain drain which argued that developing countries should not necessarily think in geographical terms, but instead keep a database of their human capacity abroad including their areas of work and availability to do consultancies in their home country. Countries could make use of such a database whenever they felt it was needed and in that way local people would keep on contributing to development in their own country.*
> — Burundi site-visit report

> *Communication is a huge challenge. The only effective means of communication with people at the district level is through radio — the walkie-talkie system. If you look, for example, at our own institute, which is internationally recognized, only the Director has access to the internet and email.*
> — Dr Soumare Absatou N'iaye, Community Health Department, Mali

Research capacity-strengthening is not only about training more researchers but also about retaining them once they are trained. Stemming the flow of researchers out of developing countries remains a significant challenge. National leadership needs to invest in health researchers as much as in health-research projects and programs. Researchers should reap rewards in recognition and remuneration. An interim solution to the brain-drain problem might be for national research-coordinating bodies to think less in geographical terms and attempt to enlist national researchers abroad to work on health problems in their home countries. Information poverty is a serious obstacle facing health researchers in the developing world. The simple lack of equipment, computers, telephones, and electricity is a major barrier.

GREATER REGIONAL COOPERATION

> *Countries need to join hands at the regional level to have a stronger voice at the global level to say that these are our problems and ensure that there is greater equity in the distribution of resources for health research.*
> — Dr Akhtar Ali Qureshi, Health Services Academy, Ministry of Health, Pakistan

> *There should be an effective African network in which research results and experiences are shared amongst African countries. This would allow those countries that are less fortunate to benefit from the results and experiences of other African countries. It will also allow for identification and recognition of the experts within Africa. ... Cooperative agreements between countries in Africa should be strengthened and harmonized so that donors cannot play countries against each other.*
> — Sudan site-visit report

> *Countries try to get donors on board at the country level, but are often unsuccessful. I would love to see a donors' meeting facilitated by COHRED for East Africa or West Africa. We need the donors' goodwill to sit down around a table, listen to country priorities and then allocate monies, say for the next three years, in these specific areas to specific countries.*
>
> — Professor Raphael Owor, Faculty of Medicine, Makerere University, Uganda

That there is "strength in numbers" is a prevailing truism, not only when comes to mobilizing external donor funding, but also when it comes to sharing research expertise. African-country representatives, in particular, perceive the need to build regional networks to give a stronger voice to country concerns at the international level. As well, those countries with fewer resources may benefit from the experience of the more fortunate ones. A regional research program would eliminate duplication of effort and the resulting waste of the region's limited resources.

A NEW DEAL WITH DONORS

> *Countries should stop their "beggar attitude" in regard to donors and realize that it is their global right to demand equity in research for health internationally.*
>
> — Sudan site-visit report

> *Africans should stop looking at global resources as charity — money which you get from the North so that you can do a few small studies here and there. Global resources are actually common resources which are available to the best scientists who can put together the best proposals to answer the most difficult questions which benefit the greatest majority of people.*
>
> — Dr Steve Chandiwana, Blair Research Institute, Ministry of Health and Child Welfare, Zimbabwe

> *International donors need to develop trust to work with countries.*
>
> — Dr Mohamed Said Abdullah, National Health Research and Development Centre, Kenya

> *The donors have double standards with respect to overhead fees, giving the developed world up to 30 percent administrative overheads and the developing world between five and 10 percent only. This should be harmonised according to an international performance output criteria.*
>
> — Sudan site-visit report

Research is a global good. Many developing countries must lose their "beggar attitude" toward international donors. By the same token, we need a new global research-funding architecture and donor mindset to allow funding to go directly to Southern researchers and institutions. Currently, a two-tier research architecture is in place that views scientists from the South as second-class researchers — "field researchers" or "national scientists." Donors channel funds through Northern institutions, and the institutions use these funds largely to support the work of their own Northern researchers, not that of their Southern "partners."

CONCLUSION

At the start of the new century, ENHR appears well poised to improve health for all, based on country-led research and action. A clearer sense of mission will guide this work, one of putting countries first, working for equity in health, and linking research to policy and action. Yet, the future demands change, not just at the country level, but at the district, regional, and global levels as well, to achieve the goals of ENHR. COHRED has emerged from its adolescent years with a keener sense of its organizational identity. In its multiple roles as advocate, broker, learning community, and collegium, it will continue to respond creatively and effectively to the needs and concerns expressed by countries.

APPENDIX 8.1
LIST OF NATIONAL RESEARCH LEADERS
AND SITE-VISIT REPORTS USED IN THE SURVEY

National research leaders

Dr Mohamed Said Abdullah
National Health Research and
    Development Centre, Kenya

Prof. Gopal Prasad Acharya
Nepal Health Research Council,
    Nepal

Dr Said Ameerberg
Mauritius Institute of Health,
    Mauritius

Dr Boungnong Bhoupa
Council of Medical Sciences
Ministry of Health, Lao PDR

Dr Steve Chandiwana
Blair Research Institute
    Ministry of Health and Child
    Welfare, Zimbabwe

Mr Abu Yusuf Choudhury
Programme for the Introduction
    and Adaption of Contraceptive
    Technology, Bangladesh

Dr Somsak Chunharas
National Institute of Health
Ministry of Public Health, Thailand

Prof. Pham Huy Dung
Centre for Social Science Research
    for Health
Ministry of Health, Viet Nam

Prof. E.M. Essien
Haematology Department
University of Ibadan, Nigeria

Dr Izzy Gerstenbluth
Department of Epidemiology
and Research
Medical and Public Health Service
of Curaçao, Curaçao

Dr Samia Yousif Idris Habbani
Research Directorate
Federal Ministry of Health, Sudan

Dr Soumare Absatou N'iaye
Community Health Department,
Mali

Prof. Raphael Owor
Faculty of Medicine
Makerere University, Uganda

Dr Michael Phillips
Research Centre of Clinical
Epidemiology
Beijing Hui Long Guan Hospital,
China

Prof. Akhtar Ali Qureshi
Health Services Academy
Ministry of Health, Pakistan

Dr Bassiouni S. Salem
Upgrading Primary Health Care
Services
Ministry of Health and Population,
Egypt

Dr Lye Munn Sann
Institute of Medical Research,
Malaysia

Dr Agus Suwandono
Center for Health Systems
Research and Development
Ministry of Health, Indonesia

Prof. Tissa Vitarana
Technology and Human Resources
Development
Ministry of Science, Sri Lanka

Site-visit reports

Benin

Burkina Faso

Burundi

Sudan

CHAPTER 9

HEALTH RESEARCH FOR DEVELOPMENT: REALITIES AND CHALLENGES

Charas Suwanwela and Victor Neufeld

SUMMARY

Summarizing the earlier chapters of this book, this concluding chapter reviews the new and not so new realities confronting the global health-research community at the beginning of the 21st century:

- *Widening disparities* — Despite some indications of progress in human development over the 1990s, health and socioeconomic disparities have widened for many countries and populations. More than 80 countries have lower per capita incomes than a decade ago, and the income gap between the richest and poorest quintiles of the world's people continues to widen, from 30 to 1 in 1960, to 60 to 1 in 1990, to 74 to 1 in 1997. With some exceptions, the health gap between countries is widening as well, particularly for three country groups: African countries suffering most severely from the AIDS epidemic, countries in Eastern and Central Europe where infrastructures have collapsed and sociobehavioural illnesses are escalating, and countries ravaged by prolonged and devastating internal conflicts. Again with some exceptions, within-country disparities in health have also widened — a phenomenon not limited to developing countries.

- *Globalization* — Even though some aspects of globalization have a long history, the past decade saw an accelerated growth in this phenomenon. Examples include new markets, new organizations (for example, the World Trade Organization [WTO]), new rules, and faster communication tools.

Some aspects of globalization do improve the conditions of the poor ("globalization with a human face"), but for the most part it has increased poverty, inequality, and insecurity. Globalization has had impacts on health, for example, through the actions of transnational corporations in the sale and control of pharmaceuticals and the marketing of tobacco in low-income countries.

— *Continuing pandemics* — Several major health conditions affecting millions of people around the world loom larger than they did a decade ago, such as the epidemic of tobacco-related diseases, accounting for perhaps 4 million deaths in 2000. Another is the AIDS epidemic — HIV-1 is now the single largest cause of death from infectious disease, expected to account for 2.5 million deaths in 2000. When measured by disability-adjusted life years (DALY), injuries (both intentional and unintentional) account for 16% of all DALY and more than 6 million deaths annually. Malaria continues to worsen, particularly in Africa.

— *Knowledge and new information and communication technologies* — Over the past decade, knowledge has become a central element in human development. Many high-income countries now call themselves "knowledge societies," reflecting the impact of the knowledge explosion on economic and social development. The new information and communication technologies (ICTs) are a major feature of this remarkable trend. Yet, the world's poorest people, 2 billion or more, are missing out on the potential benefits. Despite some promising innovations, such as the use of community-based tele-centres, large investments of money, persistence, and creativity are still needed to ensure that health knowledge improves the lives of the poor.

— *New understandings of health and development* — The development community increasingly sees health as an integral part of human development. The 1990s brought us three important insights:

- Investing in health is critical to economic productivity and human development,

- Greater equity promotes economic growth and development, and

– The application of knowledge is central to global development.

Despite the growing recognition that knowledge production and use are critical to health in development, most of the world's poor have yet to benefit from the fruits of health research. Some key challenges for the new decade are presented in this chapter, which gives special attention to the following strategic implications for the leadership of health research in low-income countries:

- *Persisting with the equity goal* — Although large and growing inequities remain, something can be done, and persisting with the equity goal is therefore critical. Strategically targeted health research can accelerate progress toward the equity goal. These strategies include focused epidemiological studies, analytic studies to explain the causes of health inequities, cost-effectiveness studies for interventions that produce the best outcomes for poor and marginalized peoples, and practical operational research to improve the use of available health interventions.

- *Strengthening national health-research systems* — The reasons for placing a major emphasis on strengthening country-specific health-research mechanisms are as valid today as they were 10 years ago, when the Commission on Health Research for Development made its strong and clear recommendations. Although many countries have made substantial progress and more tools and strategies are now available, much remains to be done, including establishing regional and global support mechanisms with a focus on the needs and realities of low-income countries.

- *Focusing on capacity development for national health-research managers* — Complex leadership competencies are needed for equity-oriented, priority-driven health research. National health-research managers may benefit from more systematic and comprehensive capacity-development programs. This chapter suggests some specific strategies to develop competencies, such as those needed to manage knowledge, create demand for research, build coalitions, and foster leadership skills among junior colleagues. These strategies include the dissemination of appropriate materials (increasingly through electronic channels) and the use of these materials in "learning-while-doing" situations, supplemented by skilled mentoring and purpose-specific events.

— *Going local* — To create a concurrent but countervailing trend to globalization, national health-research leaders must concentrate increasingly on local systems. The strategy of decentralization in health-sector reform illustrates this phenomenon. This chapter offers several suggestions for strengthening the role of research in local health development, including an emphasis on local capacity development and on equity-oriented research-to-action projects.

— *Building coalitions* — Activities in health research for development over the past decade have too often been fragmented, uncoordinated, uneven, and unsustained. The reasons are more human than technical or conceptual. Using the benefit of some promising experience, backed by scholarly studies of the coalition-building process, this chapter makes several suggestions, including the proposal that the new critical mass should be national and subnational research and learning networks that are focused on specific health problems and firmly linked to other relevant regional and global research efforts.

The chapter concludes with a call for renewed collaboration, driven by values of fairness and solidarity, and for intensified, purposeful action to ensure that health research becomes a stronger tool to improve the health of all people.

INTRODUCTION

Much of the world, perhaps 2 billion people or more, will fail to share in the benefits of global growth without a complete change in international strategy. ... A better balance needs to be struck between incentives for innovation on one hand, and the interests of the poorest on the other. ... the world's leaders have a chance to will both the ends and the means for the kind of globalisation that can serve all the world. They must seize this chance.

— Sachs (2000, p. 81)

This challenge was put to the world's leaders who met at the United Nations Millennium Assembly in September 2000. A similar challenge confronts the global health research and development community, which is now taking stock of its collective achievements of the past decade and charting a course for the future.

This final chapter begins with an overview of important new realities (some of them not so new) impacting on the global health-research community at the beginning of the 21st century, as described in previous chapters. This is followed by a summary of the major challenges these features of the global situation present to those committed to strengthening the contribution of health research to the well-being of the world's people.

NEW AND NOT SO NEW REALITIES

The dawning of a new millennium has stimulated much analysis and reflection on the human condition and the challenges ahead. These contributions can be found in the annual reports of global agencies, special editions of professional journals, and many other sources. It is a somewhat daunting task to extract the facts and insights most relevant to the aims of this book. The following list is necessarily selective, an attempt to present those aspects of the global situation that relate most directly to the goal of health research for equity in development. These new and not so new realities are

— Widening disparities;

— Globalization;

— Continuing pandemics;

— Knowledge and the new ICTs; and

— New understandings of health and development.

WIDENING DISPARITIES

In the *Human Development Report 1999*, the United Nations Development Programme (UNDP) included a balance sheet of human development, presenting some facts about human development from 1990 to 1997 (UNDP 1999). This information pertained to health, education, and other sectors and fell under two headings: global progress and global deprivation. The table in the report is a reminder that both advances and regressions occurred in the 1990s.

On the progress side of the ledger, for example, a life expectancy at birth of more than 70 years was found in 84 countries in 1997, which was up from 55 countries in 1990. Within this group of countries, the number of developing countries rose from 22 to 49. Between 1990 and 1997, the share of the population with access to safe water nearly doubled, from 40% to 72%. During the same period, adult literacy rose from 64% to 76%. Food production per capita increased by nearly 25%. The ratio of girls to boys enrolled in secondary schools increased from 36% to 61%. The decade saw these and other significant achievements.

However, from several recent sources the sobering observation is that for most developing countries and many population groups disparities widened during the past decade. Economic disparities are particularly well documented, but disparities across gender, race, and geography also widened. In the *World Development Report 1999/2000: Entering the 21st Century,* the World Bank put the following question: What has been the record to date of development? (World Bank 2000). It went on to note that some parts of the world have made gains. For example, in South Asia as a region, the proportion of the population living on less than 1 USD/day declined. But it has increased in other regions, such as Africa and Latin America. Using the commonly accepted benchmark of 3% or more as the rate of per capita growth needed to reduce poverty significantly, one finds that between 1995 and 1997 only 21 developing countries met this rate — 12 of them in Asia. Of the 48 countries designated least developed, only 6 met this benchmark. Overall, more than 80 countries now have per capita incomes lower than a decade ago. The worldwide total of those living on 1 USD/day or less continues to rise, in part because of an increase in overall population levels. From 1.2 billion in 1987, the total number of people living on this amount today is 1.5 billion. With current trends, this figure will be 1.9 billion in 2015. Another 2 billion people or more survive on 2 USD/day. The World Bank added this sobering note: "Current trends suggest that even the gains achieved could prove short-lived in the absence of new policies and institutions" (World Bank 2000, p. 24). The income gap between the fifth of the world's people living in the richest countries and the fifth living in the poorest countries continued to rise in the 1990s, from 30 to 1 in 1960, to 60 to 1 in 1990, to 74 to 1 in 1997. A startling statement from the 1999 UNDP report highlights the enormity of this income gap: "The assets of the 200 richest people are more than the combined income of 41% of the world's people. And the assets of the top three billionaires are more than the combined GNP [gross national product] of all least developed countries and their 600 million people" (UNDP 1999, p. 3).

Although health status has improved in most countries in the past decade, it appears to be worsening in some developing countries. For instance, in Kenya the infant mortality rate increased from 62 per 1 000 live births in 1993 to 74 per 1 000 live births in 1998.

The mortality rate for children under 5 years old increased from 96 per 1 000 live births to 112 per 1 000 live births during the same period. The prevalence of chronic undernutrition increased from 32.1% in 1987 to 34% in 1998. The economic crisis in Indonesia also saw an increase in the rate of children with malnutrition.

Regarding within-country health disparities, it is important to strive for a balanced assessment. In some countries, the health gap narrowed during this past decade. In a helpful annex on assessing progress, the most recent human development report illustrates the virtue of using diverse measurement perspectives (UNDP 2000). Taking immunization of infants in Egypt as an example and using an "average perspective," one sees only 67% of infants immunized in 1992, compared with 93% in 1998. Using distributional data (the "inequality perspective"), one finds that the gap in immunization rates between the best- and worst-off regions narrowed dramatically over this same 6-year period, from 31% to 7% (UNDP 2000). UNDP presented similar findings from Guatemala, comparing mortality rates between 1995 and 1998–99 for children under 5 years old. Gaps narrowed between various social groups: geographic (regional), urban–rural, and ethnic groups (UNDP 2000). But for many countries, including some high-income countries, the health gap between various population groups has widened. In the *World Health Report 1999*, the World Health Organization (WHO) gave data from around 1990 on the health status of the poor versus the nonpoor (WHO 1999). WHO's intention was to provide updated information on health inequalities on a regular basis so that comparisons over time can be made. Another sign of the importance of this topic is that the first 2000 issue of the *Bulletin of the World Health Organization* featured the theme of inequalities in health (Feachem 2000), including several national, regional, and global analyses of health disparities.

The health gap is also widening between countries. In the last several years, it has become apparent that in many countries, the health situation is in fact deteriorating. These countries fall into three groups:

- In several countries of sub-Saharan Africa, indicators show reversals in previous health gains, primarily as a result of the AIDS epidemic. For nine countries in Africa, studies project a loss of 17 years of life expectancy by 2010 — back to the levels of the 1960s. Ten years from now, in Botswana, where 36% of the adult population now has the HIV infection, the life expectancy from birth will be 29 years. In Namibia and

Zimbabwe, it will be 33 years; and in South Africa, 35 (WHO 1999).

— Researchers attribute health setbacks in some of the former socialist republics of Eastern and Central Europe to a disintegrating health and social infrastructure, along with a complex set of sociobehavioural factors.

— A third group comprises countries where the health of the population has deteriorated because of war. In Iraq, the health status, particularly of children, continues to decline, partly as a result of United Nations sanctions. Protracted within-country conflicts in places such as Afghanistan, Angola, Sierra Leone, and Sudan have had devastating consequences for the health and well-being of their citizens.

GLOBALIZATION

Much has been written about the globalization phenomenon, particularly in the last few years. Although aspects of globalization have been evident for decades — even centuries — some people nevertheless argue that certain features of it are new. In a box entitled "Globalization — What's Really New?," the *Human Development Report 1999* displayed a list of "what's new this time" (UNDP 1999, p. 30). The list included new markets, new actors (WTO, for example), new rules and norms, and faster and cheaper communication tools. Overall, the report tried to present a balanced assessment of this phenomenon ("globalization with a human face"), suggesting that societies benefit both from the free flow of money and trade and from the free flow of ideas and information (driven by new technologies). But it also recognized that globalization negatively affects marginalized groups and that it is creating new threats to several kinds of human security: financial, occupational, personal, cultural, and environmental. Global competition is putting pressure on the time, resources, and incentives for the "caring" aspect of human development, an essential element for social cohesion and strong communities. What is more, global competition is placing developing countries, which have less ability to cope and compete, in a disadvantaged position. This results in further deterioration of social and economic conditions. ICTs are creating polarization — a point that Sachs emphasized in his recent essay, "A New Map of the World" (Sachs 2000). Free flow of information also creates demands beyond the economic affordability of individuals or countries. The United Nations General Assembly vigorously debated the entire issue of globalization at its special session in Geneva in June 2000. One writer reporting on this session said that

> *The ... session concluded that poverty, inequality and insecurity have increased since globalism was launched. The time has come to write the obituary of globalism as an economic doctrine that purports to bring progress and development to international society. It has failed.*
>
> (Pfaff 2000, p. 6)

What are the impacts of globalization on health and health policy? This question raises important issues (Lee 1998; Bettcher et al. 2000). Some people express concerns about the role of transnational corporations in the control and sale of pharmaceuticals and the marketing of tobacco in developing countries. A particularly contentious issue concerns the Trade-Related Aspects of Intellectual Property Rights (TRIPs) agreement. This introduces an international standard (enforceable through WTO) to protect the intellectual property rights of the inventors and link these rights to trade. But are society's rights adequately protected? For example, many developing countries have laws to intentionally exclude pharmaceuticals from product-patent protection (allowing only process patents). The move to protect patents introduced under the TRIPs agreement limits opportunities for companies in low-income countries to produce less expensive versions of important drugs (UNDP 2000, p. 84). The General Agreement on Tariffs and Trade also exposes developing-country institutions to a more hostile world in which they cannot compete.

CONTINUING PANDEMICS

A pandemic is any health condition that causes more than 1 million deaths a year. The intention of this section is not to describe current pandemics in any detail. Many useful reports have already done so (WHO 1999). Rather, it is to use a few examples to remind the reader that pandemics are continuing; in some instances, they are much larger than they were 10 years ago. Importantly, most of these conditions disproportionately affect the poor. From this perspective, the 10-year report card of the global health community's performance (including the health-research sector) is not encouraging:

— *Tobacco-related illnesses* — Mortality and morbidity rates of illnesses caused by tobacco have continued to rise, from less than 3 million deaths annually 10 years ago to a current rate of 4 million deaths a year. Tobacco-related deaths will increase to 10 million a year by the late 2020s, and 70% of these deaths will be in developing countries (WHO 1999). We urgently need locally relevant research in support of tobacco control to convince governments, health professionals, and consumers of the risks of smoking.

- *HIV–AIDS* — Whereas HIV-1 was responsible for some 300 000 deaths in 1990, it is now the single largest cause of death from infectious disease and is expected to cause about 2.5 million deaths in 2000. This pandemic illustrates the global equity gap: 95% of the world's 34 million HIV-infected people live in developing countries, but these countries receive only 12% of the money spent on AIDS worldwide. Recently suggested research priorities for developing countries include randomized trials of behavioural interventions to prevent HIV and assessments of the cost-effectiveness of making drugs more widely available to treat opportunistic infections (Ainsworth and Waranya 2000).

- *Injuries* — Injuries account for 16% of all DALY (compared with 7% for the combination of HIV–AIDS, tuberculosis, and maternal conditions). Almost 6 million people died of injuries in 1998, more than a million from road traffic accidents. More than 2 million died from intentional injuries; almost half of these were self-inflicted. Homicide, violence, and war account for the rest. Recent research is beginning to reveal the enormity of the global burden of illness suffered by women as a result of violence (Yusuf et al. 2000). Almost twice as many war-related deaths occurred in 1998 as in 1990. All of these situations add costs in addition to human lives. The Carnegie Commission on Preventing Deadly Conflicts estimated that the cost of the seven major wars in the 1990s (not including Kosovo) to the international community was 200 billion USD — during the same period in which the flow of development aid steadily declined (UNDP 2000). Although researchers have also studied the health effects of war (Bush 2000; Spiegel and Salama 2000), we need to do much more on this topic.

- *Malaria* — Another example of a condition making the global burden of illness worse today than 10 years ago is malaria — more than 1.1 million deaths in 1998, compared with less than a million in 1990. Again, this is a condition that affects the vulnerable — particularly children and the poor, who constitute 90% of cases in sub-Saharan Africa. The economic impact of malaria in Africa is substantial:

estimated productivity losses through premature death and illness may be greater than 1% of gross national product. The challenges to the health-research community are enormous; nevertheless, it is encouraging to note evidence of increased collaboration and funding to "roll back" this disease through research and action.

The list could go on to include other major conditions. For some conditions, the global burden of illness is larger than it was 10 years ago; tuberculosis and maternal mortality are examples. For other conditions, trends in death and disability demonstrate modest progress over the 1990s; examples are the water-borne and respiratory diseases. Mental-health disorders, as a category of illness, constitute an increasingly large proportion of the illness burden, causing an estimated 10% of all DALY in low- to middle-income countries in 1998 (Ustun 2000).

KNOWLEDGE AND THE NEW ICTs

> ... *economies are built not merely through the accumulation of physical capital and human skill, but on a foundation of information, learning and adaptation. Because knowledge matters, understanding how people and societies acquire and use knowledge — and why they sometimes fail to do so — is essential to improving people's lives, especially the lives of the poorest.*
>
> — World Bank (1999, p. iii)

This is the introductory paragraph from the *World Development Report 1998/99: Knowledge for Development* (World Bank 1999). It illustrates the increasing attention paid to knowledge as a central element of human development. In fact, some propose that knowledge **is** development. The World Bank report focused on two kinds of knowledge, each with its own distinctive set of challenges. The challenge concerning "knowledge of technology" (for example, in the health or agricultural sector) is to narrow the wide gaps in social development by acquiring, absorbing, and communicating all forms of knowledge. Another kind of knowledge, that of "attributes," concerns the quality of a product or work done by an individual or institution. Knowledge of this kind can relate to problems that hurt the poor, such as when institutions fail to understand the issues confronting the poor. Solving these problems involves taking the time to learn about these people's particular needs and concerns so that they are less isolated and can improve their access to certain institutions and resources.

The debate about the evolution of the "knowledge economy" has its counterpart in the health sector. One formulation (Suwanwela 2000) suggests that the generation of knowledge (that is, research) is a product of three elements:

— Health-research planning, policy development, and management;

— Capacity development for health research; and

— Collaborative health-research programs (including the public and private sectors).

The resulting body of knowledge must then go through further processes, including

— "Optimization" (validation and meta-analysis);

— Dissemination; and

— Use (to develop policy, sustain evidence-based practices, empower people, and educate health workers).

Part of the discussion of the optimal use of available knowledge is linked to the idea of empowerment through knowledge and involves a debate about how to integrate both "scientific" knowledge and the indigenous wisdom of various societies. One approach to the bridging of the knowledge-to-action gap in the health field is "translational research" (see Box 9.1).

Fueling the "information explosion" is a remarkable increase in the availability and use of ICTs, an issue not mentioned in the 1990 Commission report. The facts are well known, and they are symbolized on the cover of the *Human Development Report 1999*: it depicts the geography of the world's Internet users in mid-1998 (UNDP 1999). At that time, 88% of Internet users lived in industrialized countries (constituting 15% of the world's population). In contrast, the 20% of the world's population living in South Asia constituted less than 1% of all Internet users. Another index is teledensity. A teledensity of 1 is one telephone for every 100 people. A quarter of the world's countries do not have even this basic level of access to telecommunications. Sweden's teledensity in 1998 was almost 70 (mainline telephones per 100 persons). Information technology is thus creating another form of global polarization and contributes to widening disparities.

Can ICTs contribute to sustainable human development, rather than detract from it? This question led to a study by the United Nations Commission on Science and Technology for Development.

> **Box 9.1**
>
> ### Translational research:
> ### Bridging the knowledge-to-action gap
>
> To date, efforts to address the gap separating knowledge from policy and action have largely taken the form of academic training and support for clinical and university-based health researchers, an approach that presupposes a seamless transition from *evidence* obtained by researchers to action taken by practitioners, policymakers, and program planners. While acknowledging the need for interdisciplinary cooperation and evidence **transfer** this approach ignores the complexity and dynamics of knowledge generation — including cross-sectoral, cross-contextual, and cross-cultural reasoning and participatory processes — all of which are part of evidence **translation**. It also overlooks the experiential evidence and expertise present in businesses, communities, governments, and nongovernmental organizations.
>
> It is time to extend the meaning of *evidence*, argues Dr Dennis Willms (McMaster University, Hamilton, Ontario, Canada), beyond the results of traditional academic or scientific research to a broader definition encompassing experiential, intuitive, spiritual, practical, and expert knowledge. Such a definition would facilitate the involvement of multiple stakeholders in a participatory process of dialogue and negotiation to arrive at a shared framework for understanding and seeking solutions to priority health problems.
>
> This participatory process is a defining feature of what he calls **translational research**. Translational research entails the systematic eliciting of, and building on, evidential and experiential stories from a wide range of stakeholders. The many actors engage in a process of structured reflection and action. Intentionally organized forums provide an opportunity for sharing understandings of the determinants of, and evidence for, a specific health problem, agreeing on a mutual language for framing these understandings and negotiating joint solutions. Referred to as "conceptual events" by Willms, these forums give equal time and voice to dissonant perspectives. They have the potential to form the basis for the design, dissemination, and evaluation of health interventions that are equitable, sustainable, culturally appropriate, and psychologically compelling.
>
> Source: Based on an interview with Dr Willms.

The report of this inquiry is now available as a source book (Mansell and Wehn 1998). Its central conclusion is that "ICTs can make a major contribution to sustainable development but that this opportunity will be accompanied by major risks" (Mansell and Wehn 1998, p. 256). The report went on to say that developing countries would need to invest in two kinds of capabilities — technological and "social" (that is, the ability to use ICTs). We can expect greater returns from investments in enhancing utilization capabilities.

Health-research managers in developing countries are often well aware of the exciting prospects that the advances in ICTs offer in facilitating health-research development. Many have seen the benefits first hand, during their training in industrialized countries or other international exchanges. Some leaders of national health-research institutions envision ICTs serving as a bridge between the global world of knowledge and the specific information needs of research groups, policymakers, and the general public in developing countries. However, a host of constraints prevent their realizing this vision, including inadequate funding, weak infrastructures, an ongoing brain drain, and low levels of research uptake. Creative means must be found through international partnerships to reduce the interaction costs of knowledge management. These strategies would include enhancement of the capacities of support staff, free access to international electronic journals, and direct opportunities for research managers to acquire ICT skills. Horton (2000) recently offered some useful insights into the role of researchers, editors, and publishers. We can add to such practical measures by creating and facilitating local learning and innovative coalitions (as suggested in Chapter 4).

NEW UNDERSTANDINGS OF HEALTH AND DEVELOPMENT

Copenhagen Plus Five, a special session of the United Nations, convened in Geneva in June 2000, five years after the 1995 World Summit for Social Development. WHO's submission to this follow-up meeting makes the case that health is both an input and an outcome of development. The argument is as follows:

> *If health is an asset and ill-health a liability for poor people, protecting and promoting health are central to the entire process of poverty eradication and human development. As such they should be goals of development policy shared by all sectors — economic, environmental and social.*
> (WHO 2000a, p. 7)

The WHO document puts forward three action proposals as integral elements of the Copenhagen Plus Five follow-up plan:

— Strengthen global policy for social development;

— Integrate health dimensions into social and economic policy; and

— Develop health systems to meet the needs of poor and vulnerable populations.

These proposals illustrate an increasing confidence among health planners as they and the development community discuss the importance of health in human development. It has led some to put forward the idea of "health-led development," arguing that health improvements and economic growth are mutually reinforcing, both positively and negatively (Bloom and Canning 2000). The Nobel Laureate economist Amartya Sen provided a more focused analysis (Sen 1999b). Agreeing that "good health is an *integral part* of good development," he went on to argue that low-income countries should use "support-led" processes, focused strategically on more health care, education, and other social programs (Sen 1999b, p. 623). WHO's Commission on Macroeconomics and Health, launched in January 2000, is studying the links between health and economic growth in more depth. One of the six issues on this commission's agenda is "the economics of investing in the research and development of drugs and vaccines primarily for poor populations" (WHO 2000b, p. 275).

Investments in research and interventions aimed at the sociobehavioural aspects of health promotion and prevention are also important. Primary and secondary prevention of many more illnesses is now possible, as a result of improved understanding of disease risk factors and their interaction. Curative technologies have advanced, becoming sophisticated, as well as costly. The increased demand for specialized care adds to the challenges confronting health-care systems. The public sector can no longer take sole responsibility for provision of care — promotive, preventive, or curative. Financing schemes and business investments in health-care provision under market conditions need appropriate regulatory and consumer-protection mechanisms. Education and mass media play important roles in the new health system. In many instances, the limited resources available to individuals or countries are drawn to the less productive and less cost-effective part of the health-care system. Health development as a whole is affected. Research on the economic and management aspects of health-care systems is therefore also greatly needed.

The author of Chapter 3, David Harrison, takes the argument a step further by considering health research in the context of three important insights from the 1990s:

- Investing in health is critical to economic productivity and human development;

- Greater equity promotes economic growth and human development; and
- The application of knowledge is central to global development.

Thus, research (knowledge production) is not only a strategic tool for making improvements in health but also a "driving force behind all development" (Harrison, this volume, p. 48). Some preliminary explorations in "mapping" the relationship between health research and development are offered in Figure A3.1. Despite this theoretical underpinning, however, the reality is that, because of the market forces of globalization, coupled with narrow scientific incentives, the world has diverted knowledge-related human and financial resources away from the concerns of the poor in low-income countries.

CHALLENGES IN HEALTH RESEARCH FOR DEVELOPMENT FOR THE NEXT DECADE

Some compelling reasons are described above to view health research as, potentially, "an essential link to equity in development," as envisioned in the title of the 1990 Commission report. People in the development community increasingly regard knowledge production and use as critical elements of health in developing countries. Yet, most of the world's poor have yet to benefit from the fruits of health research. This chapter highlights five challenges for the coming decade. All these challenges derive from earlier chapters, and we restate them here to emphasize their importance:

- Persisting with the equity goal;
- Strengthening national health-research systems;
- Focusing on capacity development of national health-research managers;
- Going local; and
- Building coalitions.

With each challenge, we explore some strategic implications for national health-research systems for the attention of the national leaders and people responsible for regional and global support mechanisms.

PERSISTING WITH THE EQUITY GOAL

As stated in a special issue of the *Bulletin of the World Health Organization* on inequalities in health, an inequity is an unfair and remediable inequality (Feachem 2000). As described above, large and growing inequities remain. But something can be done about them. Thus, the first and overarching challenge is simply and clearly to persist with the equity goal and make health research contribute more effectively to achieving this goal.

The reasons for persisting with this goal are the following (COHRED 2000e):

— The determinants of health status should not be socioeconomic status or any other social distinction, such as gender, ethnicity, age, or geography;

— Equity-oriented development strategies contribute directly to economic growth and human development;

— Concentrating health investments on those who carry the largest disease burden (usually the poor and marginalized groups) improves efficiency; and

— Relatively small investments in the application of existing knowledge can result in substantial health gains for disadvantaged groups (practical operational [problem-solving] research can improve the efficient application of available and affordable health interventions).

At the country level, strategically targeted health research can accelerate progress toward the equity goal. Epidemiological studies can pinpoint inequities in health status. Analytic studies can provide explanations for existing inequities. Cost-effectiveness research can identify those interventions that produce the greatest desired outcomes for poor and marginalized groups. Carefully selected and applied monitoring tools can determine progress in achieving the health-equity goal. These and other equity-oriented research strategies are most practical at the subnational (community) level.

Health research can no longer be exclusively the domain of researchers. It needs to be demystified and made understandable to other stakeholders. For too long, the demand side of health research has been less emphasized than the supply side. The capacity of research users must be strengthened so they can take a more active part in applying research results to health problems. Policymakers can demonstrate accountability and evidence-based decision-making by participating more fully in the research process. Similarly, research can assist policy implementers with technology assessment, operational choices, and evaluation. Individuals and communities learn to ask the right questions and assess alternative answers when they are involved in research. Indeed, being able to do health research for themselves empowers developing countries in their health planning and provision of care.

STRENGTHENING NATIONAL HEALTH-RESEARCH SYSTEMS

Several developing countries have followed the example of high-income countries in deriving economic and social benefits from investing in the generation of new knowledge or from adapting existing knowledge to national purposes (World Bank 1999). The reasons given in the 1990 Commission report for the focus on national health research remain valid to this day. But progress has been slow and fragmented. The message from research leaders in low-income countries is consistent: the overall strategy is correct, but much remains to be done (see Chapter 8). Several chapters in this book provide specific suggestions to strengthen national health-research systems, including

— Investing scarce resources more efficiently (Chapter 3);

— Enhancing community participation (Chapter 4);

— Linking the research and policy processes more effectively (Chapter 5); and

— Broadening capacity-strengthening strategies to include national networks (forums), in addition to focusing on individuals and organizations (Chapter 6).

It is also important to understand the dynamic interconnectivity of levels: global, regional, national, and subnational. For example, regional health-research organizations should, for the most part, align their agendas and activities with national research needs and perspectives, as described in Chapter 7. The same principle applies to global agencies and institutions. We can learn much more about how to develop the most effective and mutually beneficial interactions among the various levels.

Many countries have successfully established a more coordinated, priority-driven system of health research. However, significant barriers remain. One is the challenge of moving from the identification of national health-research priorities to the actual implementation of research programs and investments. Recent work in Tanzania provides some useful ideas, tools, and strategies for deploying limited resources to meet country-specific needs equitably and efficiently (Harrison 2000). Another common barrier is the lack of coordination of the inputs (technical assistance and funding) of several donors within a single country. Here a role may be possible for a more explicit "bridging" and coalition-building of the national health-research leadership with external partners, such as the Council on Health Research for Development (COHRED) or a bilateral agency.

FOCUSING ON CAPACITY DEVELOPMENT OF NATIONAL HEALTH-RESEARCH MANAGERS

In practical terms, the day-to-day work of innovation and change depends on people being determined to make a difference, individually and in teams. Given the emphasis of this book on the national perspective, we believe that research managers have special roles to play in guiding equity-oriented, priority-driven national health research. These people often find themselves taking on major leadership and management roles, based on seniority or a strong scientific track record, but they may be unprepared for the broader set of tasks before them. Of course, many acquire some of the required competencies informally. Our recommendation in this chapter is to take a more intentional and systematic approach to the capacity development of national health-research managers.

The definition of a *national health-research manager* can be broad enough to include those who lead the institutions that produce research as well as those that use it. In the former group are national health-research organizations, forums, networks, and other research centres. The mission of academic institutions includes both the production and the use of research, in particular the education of health professionals who will do research and use it in the future. Research-user institutions include government agencies (for example, policy and planning units of ministries), major implementation programs, and national nongovernmental organizations (NGOs). NGOs are playing an increasingly important role in the development process, at both national and global levels (Fowler 1997). Some are active in both the generation and the use of health research. Improvement in the management of health research in countries needs certain competencies that have also been identified as Essential National Health Research (ENHR) competencies: advocacy and promotion, establishing a coordinating mechanism, priority-setting, capacity development, resource mobilization, networking, and evaluation.

Chapter 6 makes some suggestions on the special competencies of national health-research managers (in addition to those attributes needed for leadership of any organization). These special competencies are as follows:

— *Knowledge management* — understanding the nature of the knowledge economy and facilitating access to global knowledge to solve local problems;

— *Demand creation* — working with user groups to accelerate the use of evidence in policy development, practice, and action;

— *Coalition-building* — using special skills to foster team-building and network development and management; and

— *Leadership development per se* — being familiar with the scholarly work on leadership and applying this in practice, such as through systematic succession planning and the mentoring of junior colleagues.

Some agencies and organizations already offer courses and workshops on health management and leadership. The reading materials in those courses focus on the role of health-research management (IDRC and WHO 1992). But more can be done to address the specific needs of national health-research managers, such as the following:

— Assemble available materials and make them accessible through "electronic libraries" (as well as "physical" libraries), perhaps in a series of learning modules — for example, a variety of assessment and conceptual tools, collections of case studies and best practices, book reviews, and annotated bibliographies.

— Combine the use of materials (as above) with systematic learning-while-doing arrangements — a strong case can be made for firmly linking the acquisition of new competencies to actual tasks and real-life problems. Managers can acquire new knowledge and skills on site, provided they have a systematic plan, time to devote, available and relevant materials, and skilled mentoring. It is particularly helpful to integrate this study into performance-assessment and quality-improvement strategies.

– Use specific events (workshops, seminars, courses) to serve as adjuncts — but they should serve as component elements of a learning program rooted in actual practice.

Two other groups, in addition to research managers, should receive special attention. One is the "emerging leaders," that is, young colleagues who have completed their formal training and have embarked on promising professional careers. They have special needs and struggles, such as balancing professional aspirations with commitments to young families and personal (nonprofessional) interests. They also require guidance and mentoring on career planning and professional development. Students are the second group — the thousands of energetic, motivated, and intelligent future health professionals studying in universities and training colleges and postgraduate programs. They are the next generation of leaders in all aspects of research: production, use, and management. Much more can be done to involve students in various aspects of research, although many training institutions already have arrangements for doing this.

Developing countries should consider the creation of explicit capacity-development programs to meet the needs of various research managers. These programs may include a component focused on emerging leaders. Regional mechanisms and global agencies may consider creating special funds and resources to facilitate this aspect of national capacity development.

GOING LOCAL — INCREASING THE EMPHASIS ON SUBNATIONAL RESEARCH SYSTEMS

The *World Development Report 1999/2000* discusses the development landscape of the first years of the 21st century (World Bank 2000). The discussion revolves around two major features of this landscape — globalization and localization. Both have their strengths and drawbacks, but both realities of our changing world have important implications for equity-oriented health research. We discussed the issue of globalization earlier, and the suggestion here is that localization presents some special challenges and opportunities for translating research into action. Strong features of localization include enhanced possibilities for community involvement in planning and local governance; also, local arrangements can be more responsive to needs (those of poor and marginalized groups, for example) and opportunities. This is illustrated in the trend toward increased decentralization as a feature of health-sector reform. However, without local capacity development and resources, decentralization can be frustrating and ineffective.

The health-development field already has a strong tradition of local action, such as the Healthy Cities initiative and Community-Oriented Primary Care. The work of most health NGOs focuses on community-based activities. For many years, WHO has been a champion of district health-system development. So a considerable base of experience is already in place.

How can we strengthen the role of research in local health development? Again, one can draw on some important experience, some of which is described in Chapter 6. The Matlab project in Bangladesh is a long-standing example of this concept (Aziz and Moseley 1997). The Navrongo field site in northern Ghana is another (Binka et al. 1995). Through systematic and sustained demographic and health surveillance, many field-site projects have contributed substantially to health-sector reform (Tollman and Zwi 2000). Several field-site projects in low- to middle-income countries have recently come together to form the International Network for Demographic Evaluation of Populations and Their Health. An Africa-based COHRED initiative is exploring the application of the ENHR strategy in district development (COHRED 1998). The University Partnerships Project (an initiative of the International Development Research Centre) explores the role of academic institutions as partners with communities and local governments in locally relevant health research. It features the active involvement of students (IDRC 1991).

The challenge is to greatly accelerate local partnerships in which all aspects of research become integral components of local health-development activities. A strategic focus can be at the district level because in many countries districts are an increasingly important geopolitical entity. Some specific elements of district-based health research are the following:

— Working within a broad development framework (consistent with the concept of health as an integral part of development) — in many cases, this means working directly and intersectorally with district development teams. National human development reports now regularly appear for many countries and provide helpful analyses and information on district development (UNDP 1999).

— Ensuring a strong capacity-building element, including all the elements of the research process, such as problem identification, priority-setting, and research use. This can be part of an ongoing process of problem-solving and district development (TEHIP News 1999).

— Putting a priority on equity-oriented research-to-action projects, including direct involvement of poor and marginalized groups.

People responsible for the mechanisms that coordinate national health research should give special attention to linking national health-research resources to district development. One way of doing this would be to create an inventory of agencies and organizations (including external agencies) conducting projects in particular districts. Some countries have also established training programs for district health managers in such areas as information management, evidence-based planning, and other relevant topics.

BUILDING COALITIONS — AN ESSENTIAL STRATEGY FOR THE 21ST CENTURY

My own view is that we are seeing the emergence of a new, much less formal structure of global governance, where governments and partners in civil society, the private sector and others are forming functional coalitions across geographic borders and traditional political lines to move public policy in ways that meet the aspirations of a global citizenry.

— UNDP (1999, p. v)

This was written by Mark Malloch Brown in the foreword to the *Human Development Report 1999*, soon after he became the new coordinator of UNDP. Under the last challenge of this chapter, we put forward the proposition that building and maintaining coalitions must be a key strategy.

Why this emphasis on coalitions? On reviewing the track record of the initiatives of the past decade, we discovered the pervading and serious criticism that these efforts have been fragmented, uncoordinated, uneven, and unsustained. This is a problem at all levels. The causes of fragmentation and lack of coordination are complex, although most observers agree that they are not primarily technical or conceptual — they are human. Individuals and organizations find it easier to protect their "turf" than to share resources and find it easier to maintain the status quo than to initiate change. But the world around us is rapidly changing, and now many of the problems of 10 years ago are larger and more pervasive.

To be balanced in our assessment, however, we should note the encouraging examples of coalition-building occurring at various levels:

- Copenhagen Plus Five brought together all the relevant United Nations agencies, the World Bank, and the International Monetary Fund to critically review progress on the global goals of social development.

- The last few years have seen an increasing number of global public–private partnerships in the health sector (Buse and Walt [2000a, 2000b] recently described and analyzed these collaborative initiatives).

- COHRED is a mechanism at the global level that responds to the needs of countries attempting to address inequities through health research. Realization of the need for appropriate tools and methodologies for the management of health research at the national and subnational levels has led to a compilation of experiences and lessons learned in various countries.

- At the regional level as well, there are many networks and collaborative arrangements related to health research, such as the Alliance for Health Policy and Services Research. It recently brought together six networks from Africa and Asia, all of them concerned with health-systems and policy research (WHO 2000c).

- At the national level, several national health-research networks or forums have recently been created (some are described in Chapter 6).

As experience with coalitions begins to build, some scholarly studies are becoming available on the various kinds of collaboration and the determinants of their effectiveness. Based on analyses of costs and benefits for participating entities, some of these studies have distinguished various forms of collaboration, such as networks, alliances, consortiums, coalitions, and coordination arrangements (Fowler 1997). Others have offered typologies of partnerships (Kickbush and Quick 1998). The most recent world development report described purpose-specific *institutions* (a broader term than organizations), which reflects the importance of policies and processes in the new development paradigm (World Bank 2000).

Cooperation among coalition members is essential to allowing for more effective and efficient partnership at several levels. For example,

— A forum where stakeholders with diverse missions, objectives, and modes of operation can talk to each other would promote better understanding and harmonization of activities, thus benefiting all; and

— Collaborative efforts and select initiatives can be launched by those stakeholders with a common interest.

Cooperation is most likely to occur when all stakeholders perceive each other as equal partners and demonstrate mutual respect. Prescriptive, domineering, and imposing views must be avoided, and differences must be reconciled. Efficiency and a common goal should dictate coordination of efforts, and a code of good practice and ethical standards for international cooperation needs to be developed. Lastly, the equity goal should always be kept in focus.

This is not the place to give a detailed analysis of coalitions and their variants. Rather, our intention is to describe the challenge, squarely before us, of doing much better than in the past in sharing information on common objectives, coordinating our efforts (to avoid wasteful duplication), and creating specific joint initiatives (coalitions, partnerships) that benefit all partners.

The following are some suggestions to be considered by national leadership teams:

— Identify coalition-building as a specific "competence," which can be described in more detail, learned, and assessed;

— Create local (national and subnational) equity-oriented health and development coalitions (as described above), with research as an integral component; and

— Engage in more systematic research on the determinants of effective coalitions and disseminate the results of such investigations.

CONCLUSION

In the final analysis, the response to the realities and challenges described in this chapter depends on the actions of individuals, those us of who work in one way or another within the global health-research system. And our actions are driven by our fundamental values. The underlying values of this book are equity and fairness — a belief in the worth of every individual and a belief that every person should have opportunities to realize their worth. This book is also about solidarity and collaboration as key requirements for achieving our goal. The goal is clear — to improve the health of all people, using health research as an essential tool. To all of this, we add a note of urgency — the challenges are immense, and there is much work to do. This is the time for renewing collaborative and purposeful efforts to meet these challenges.

APPENDIX 1

CONTRIBUTING AUTHORS

Somsak Chunharas
Dr Somsak Chunharas graduated from the Faculty of Medicine, Ramathibodi Hospital, Mahidol University in 1997. He also holds a Masters Degree in Public Health in Development and Planning from the Royal Tropical Institute, Amsterdam (1983), and a Certificate in Financing Health Care in Developing Countries from Boston University (1988). He is currently the Director of the Bureau of Health Policy and Planning of the Ministry of Public Health, Thailand. His current fields of interest are hospital management in rural Thai communities, policy analysis for health services and human-resource development, information-systems development, research management, and international health affairs. Dr Chunharas's previous appointments include those of Vice-chair of the Rural Doctor Association, Secretary-General of the Thai Medical Council, Vice President of the National Epidemiology Board of Thailand, and member of the King Ananthamahidol Foundation Medical Committee. Dr Chunharas chairs the Council for Health Research and Development Working Group on Research to Action and Policy and coordinates the Asia–Pacific Network on Health Systems and Policy Research.

Tessa Tan-Torres Edejer
Dr Tessa Tan-Torres Edejer is an internist and infectious-disease specialist from the University of the Philippines, Manila. She received training in clinical epidemiology and clinical economics through the International Clinical Epidemiology Network. Her research interests include tuberculosis, quality of care, and economic evaluations. In Manila, she has worked closely with the Essential National Health Research program in the Department of Health and with the

Tuklas-Lunas Foundation, a nongovernmental organization that supports Essential National Health Research in the Philippines. At present, she is working as a medical officer and scientist in Geneva with the World Health Organization, in the cluster of Evidence and Information for Policy.

David Harrison
David Harrison (MBChB, MSc [medicine], MPP) is currently the National Programmes Director of Lovelife, a national AIDS-prevention program in South Africa. He was the founding Executive Director of the Health Systems Trust, a nongovernmental organization supporting health-sector reform in South Africa, and subsequently directed the Initiative for Sub-District Support (aimed at improving service delivery by focusing on the quality of local health care). He chairs the Council on Health Research for Development Working Group on Promotion, Advocacy and Country Mechanisms for Essential National Health Research.

Javid Hashmi
Dr Javid Hashmi is a Fellow of the Royal College of Physicians (Edinburgh). He is a Pakistani physician who, before joining the World Health Organization (WHO) in 1979, held clinical and research appointments in Pakistan, including Director of Pakistan Medical Research Council. In WHO, he successively served as Regional Adviser of Research Promotion and Development and as Director of Health Protection and Promotion in the WHO Regional Office for the Eastern Mediterranean, followed by appointments as Chief of Research Capability Strengthening in the WHO–United Nations Development Programme–World Bank Special Programme for Research and Training in Tropical Diseases and as WHO Representative in Iran.

Nancy Johnson
Nancy Johnson (MA) is a health social scientist who works as a consultant on qualitative-research design, data collection and analysis, and development of health and social-science manuscripts. Previous research projects span a broad range of areas, including the design of culturally appropriate AIDS educational interventions in Zimbabwe; community-based maternal- and child-health programs for Latin American immigrants in Hamilton, Canada; patient-centred breast-cancer treatment decision-making; and decisions to withdraw life support in intensive-care settings. Ms Johnson also coedited *Nurtured by Knowledge: Learning to Do Participatory Action–Research* (IDRC, 1997).

Tamas Koos
Dr Koos is a graduate of Semmelweis University of Medicine, Budapest. He is currently a consultant in the area of primary health care and development.

Peter Makara
Dr Peter Makara is a social scientist from Hungary, where he has pursued his interests in health promotion and education. He was active in promoting Essential National Health Research in Hungary and Eastern Europe and joined the Board of the Council on Health Research for Development in 1999. Recently, he joined the World Health Organization European Centre for Health Policy, in Copenhagen, Denmark.

Abdelhay Mechbal
Dr Mechbal is Regional Advisor for Research and Policy Coordination for the World Health Organization Regional Office for the Eastern Mediterranean, which is in Alexandria, Egypt.

Mutuma Mugambi
Mutuma Mugambi (MD, PhD) is Professor at and Vice-Chancellor of Kenya Methodist University. He is a past Director of Medical Research in Kenya and has served as an advisor to a number of international and regional research bodies. Recently, Dr Mugambi led the African consultation to prepare for the upcoming conference on health research for development in Bangkok.

Victor Neufeld
Victor Neufeld is a physician, educator, and international consultant based in Hamilton, Canada, where he is Professor Emeritus of Medicine and Epidemiology at McMaster University. Over a period of more than 25 years, he has held various academic leadership positions in the university, the last of which was Director of the Centre for International Health. He has served as a consultant and adviser to many international agencies, institutions, and organizations in the area of capacity-building for health-system reform and leadership development.

Yvo Nuyens
Yvo Nuyens (PhD) is the Coordinator of the Council on Health Research for Development. His past appointments include Chair of the Department of Sociology and President of the Sociological Research Institute at the University of Louvain (Belgium) and

Programme Director for Health Systems Research and Development, World Health Organization Headquarters in Geneva, Switzerland. He has published a number of books and articles on the interface between health research and decision-making and on sociocultural perspectives on health and medicine.

Alberto Pellegrini Filho

Alberto Pellegrini Filho (MD, PhD) is currently Coordinator of the Research Program, Division of Health and Human Development, the World Health Organization Regional Office for the Americas and Pan American Health Organization (PAHO). Dr Pellegrini's scientific background is in neuroscience, and since joining PAHO in 1986 he has been studying and publishing on the health-research situation and policies in Latin America and the Caribbean.

David Picou

Dr David Picou is the Director of Research of the Caribbean Health Research Council (a regional organization that advises 18 Caribbean governments on all matters relating to health research). He is the Focal Point (coordinator) for Essential National Health Research (ENHR) in the Caribbean and has had some association with the Council on Health Research for Development for several years. He was Professor of Experimental Medicine and Director of the Tropical Metabolism Research Unit, Jamaica, where he worked for more than 20 years on malnutrition in infants. His continuing interests have been promotion of ENHR, health-research capacity-strengthening, and health-research ethics.

Chitr Sitthi-amorn

Chitr Sitthi-amorn (MD, PhD) is the President-elect of the International Epidemiology Association and the founding Dean of the College of Public Health, Chulalongkorn University, in Bangkok. He has a very diverse background, starting his career as a neuroscientist, then becoming a clinician, an epidemiologist, a clinical epidemiologist, and finally, the founding Dean of the College of Public Health at the oldest university in Thailand. As the Asian Focal Point (coordinator) for Essential National Health Research, he has used a combination of face-to-face meetings and electronic dialogue to capture the "Asian voice" on health research for development. He is a former member of the Board of the International Clinical Epidemiology Network and has worked with colleagues around the world in setting priorities for curriculum change, policy development, and capacity-strengthening for medicine and public health.

Charas Suwanwela

Dr Charas Suwanwela is Professor Emeritus of Medicine and former President of Chulalongkorn University. Currently, he serves as Chair of the Board of the Council on Health Research for Development, the Policy Board of the Thailand Research Promotion Fund, and the Higher Education Committee of the Thailand Ministry of University Affairs. He is a former member of the Thailand National Legislative Assembly and Senate. He received the award for Citizen of Outstanding Achievement from the National Cultural Commission of Thailand and the Distinguished Citizen Award from the Prem Tinasulanond Foundation of Thailand.

Susan Reynolds Whyte

Susan Reynolds Whyte (PhD) is Professor at the Institute of Anthropology, University of Copenhagen. She has carried out ethnographic fieldwork for many years in Kenya, Tanzania, and Uganda. In addition to publishing articles and book chapters on gender, development, and health, she coedited a book on pharmaceuticals in developing countries and one on disability and culture. Her book, *Questioning Misfortune* (Cambridge University Press, 1997) examines the management of illness and death in eastern Uganda. She has a strong interest in applied anthropology, is a member of the Board of the Council on Health Research for Development, and works with the Enhancement of Research Capacity program, funded by Danish International Development Assistance.

APPENDIX 2

ABBREVIATIONS AND ACRONYMS

ACHR	Advisory Committee on Health Research [WHO]
ACMR	Advisory Committee on Medical Research [WHO]
ARCH	Applied Research on Child Health project
ASEAN	Association of Southeast Asian Nations
BRAC	Bangladesh Rural Advancement Committee
CAB	Community Advisory Board [Trinidad and Tobago]
CARIN	Central Asian Research Information Network
CARK	Central Asian republics and Kazakhstan
CCH	Caribbean Cooperation in Health initiative
CCMRC	Commonwealth Caribbean Medical Research Council
CEEC–NIS	Central and Eastern European countries and newly independent states
CEU	clinical-epidemiological unit
CGIAR	Consultative Group on International Agricultural Research
CHRC	Caribbean Health Research Council
CMRH	Conference of Ministers Responsible for Health [Caribbean]
COHRED	Council on Health Research for Development
CONICYT	Comisión Nacional de Investigación Científica y Tecnológica (national council for scientific and technological research)
DALY	disability-adjusted life years
ENHR	Essential National Health Research
EQUINET	Southern African Regional Network on Equity in Health
GDP	gross domestic product

GFHR	Global Forum for Health Research
GNP	gross national product
GTZ	Gesellschaft für Technische Zusammenarbeit (agency for technical cooperation)
HFA/2000	Health for All by the Year 2000 [WHO]
HNP	health, nutrition, and population
HRP	Special Programme of Research, Development and Research Training in Human Reproduction
HSR	health-systems research
HST	Health Systems Trust
IAVI	International AIDS Vaccine Initiative
ICTs	information and communication technologies
IDB	Inter-American Development Bank
IDRC	International Development Research Centre
IHPP	International Health Policy Program
IMF	International Monetary Fund
INCLEN	International Clinical Epidemiology Network
ISDS	Initiative for Sub-District Support
ISSP	Immunobiologicals Self-Sufficiency Program
LDCs	least-developed countries
MIM	Multilateral Initiative on Malaria
MOH	Ministry of Health [Burkina Faso]
NAID	Norwegian Agency for International Development
NGO	nongovernmental organization
NPCB	National Programme for Control of Blindness [India]
OECD	Organisation for Economic Co-operation and Development
PAHO	Pan American Health Organization
PANSRI	Panay Self-Reliance Institute [Philippines]
PRIMA	Partage de risques maladie
R&D	research and development
S&T	science and technology
SAREC	Swedish Agency for Research Cooperation with Developing Countries
SCI	Science Citation Index

ABBREVIATIONS AND ACRONYMS

SCRPDC	Swiss Commission for Research Partnerships with Developing Countries
SEACLEN	Southeast Asia Clinical Epidemiology Network
SEAMEO	Southeast Asian Ministers of Education Organization
SIDA	Swedish International Development Agency
TDR	Special Programme for Research and Training in Tropical Diseases
TEHIP	Tanzania Essential Health Intervention Project
TRIPs	Trade-Related Aspects of Intellectual Property Rights
TROPMED	Tropical Medicine and Public Health Center [SEAMEO]
UNDP	United Nations Development Programme
UNHRO	Uganda National Health Research Organization
USD	United States dollars
VHL	Virtual Health Library [PAHO]
WHA	World Health Assembly
WHO	World Health Organization [United Nations]
WTO	World Trade Organization

APPENDIX 3

BIBLIOGRAPHY

Acemoglu, D. 1997. Training and innovation in an imperfect labor market. Review of Economic Studies, 64, 445–464.
ACHR (Advisory Committee on Health Research). 1986. Health research strategy. World Health Organization, Geneva, Switzerland. WHO/RPD/ACHR(HRS)/86.
———— 1997. A research policy agenda for science and technology to support global health development: a synopsis. World Health Organization, Geneva, Switzerland. WHO/RPS/ACHR/97.3.
Aday, L.; Begley, C.; Lairson, D.; Slater, C. 1998. Equity: concepts and methods. In Aday, L.; Begley, C.; Lairson, D.; Slater, C., ed., Evaluating the health care system: effectiveness, efficiency and equity (2nd ed.). Health Administration Press, Chicago, IL, USA. pp. 173–245.
ADDR (Applied Diarrheal Disease Research project). 1996. Linking applied research with health policy: proceedings of an international workshop. 25–28 Feb 1996, Cuernevaca, Mexico. ADDR, Boston, MA, USA.
Ad Hoc Committee (Ad Hoc Committee on Health Research Relating to Future Internvention Options). 1996. Investing in health research and development. World Health Organization, Geneva, Switzerland. TDR/Gen/96.1.
Adjei, S.; Gyapong, J. 1999. Evolution of health research essential for development in Ghana. Council on Health Research for Development, Geneva, Switzerland. Document No. 99.3.
Ainsworth, M.; Waranya, T. 2000. Breaking the silence: setting realistic priorities for AIDS control in less-developed countries. The Lancet, 356, 55–60.
Akhtar, T. 2000. Health research capacity in Pakistan. Paper presented at the WHO Meeting on Research Capacity Strengthening in Developing Countries, 26–28 Apr, Fondation Marcel Mérieux, Les Pensières, Annecy, France. World Health Organization, Geneva, Switzerland.
Alesina, A.; Rodrik, D. 1994. Distributive policies and economic growth. Quarterly Journal of Economics, 109, 465–490.

Altimir, O. 1994. Income distribution and poverty through crisis and adjustment. CEPAL Review, 52, 7–31.
Alvendia, A. 1985. A policy framework. In Silveira, M., ed., Research and development: linkages to production in developing countries. Westview Press, Boulder, CO, USA.
Amabik, T. 1999. How to kill creativity. In Harvard business review on breakthrough thinking. Harvard University, Cambridge, MA, USA.
Andersson, N. 1996. Evidence-based planning: the philosophy and methods of sentinel community surveillance. Economic Development Institute, World Bank, Washington, DC, USA.
Aziz, K.; Moseley, W. 1997. The history, methodology and main findings of the Matlab project in Bangladesh. In das Gupta, M. et al., ed., Prospective community studies in developing countries. Clarendon Press, Oxford, UK. pp. 28–53.

Baguioro, L. 1999. Kidneys for sale: a furor over the growing trade in human organs. Newsweek International (Nov), p. 54.
Baskerville, R.; Pries-Heje, J. 1997. IT diffusion and innovation models: the conceptual domains. In McMaster, T.; Mumford, E.; Swanson, E.; Warboys, B.; Wastell D., ed., Facilitating technology transfer through partnership: learning from practice and research. Chapman and Hall, London, UK.
Batangan, D.; Ujano-Batangan, T. 1999. Study on community participation in Essential National Health Research (ENHR) process: the Philippine experience. Report for COHRED's Working Group on Community Participation. Tuklas Pangkalasugan Foundation; ENHR Program, Department of Health, Philippines.
Beattie, P.; Renshaw, M.; Davies, C. 1999. Strengthening health research in the developing world: malaria research capacity in Africa. Wellcome Trust, London, UK.
Bénabou, R. 1996. Equity and efficiency in human capital investment: the local connection. Review of Economic Studies, 63, 237–264.
Berg, E. 1993. Rethinking technical cooperation: reforms for capacity building in Africa. Regional Bureau for Africa, United Nations Development Programme; Development Alternatives, Inc., New York, NY, USA.
Bettcher, D.; Yach, D.; Guindon, E. 2000. Global trade and health: key linkages and future challenges. Bulletin of the World Health Organization, 78(4), 521–534.
Bhagavan, M. 1992. The SAREC model: institutional cooperation and the strengthening of national research capacity in developing countries. Swedish Agency for Research Cooperation with Developing Countries, Stockholm, Sweden.
Binka, F.; Nazzar, A.; Phillips, J. 1995. The Navrongo Community Health and Family Planning Project. Studies in Family Planning, 26(3), 121–139.

Birdsall, N.; Jaspersen, F., ed. 1997. Pathways to growth: comparing East Asia and Latin America. Inter-American Development Bank, Washington, DC, USA.

Birdsall, N.; Rhee, C. 1993. Does R&D contribute to economic growth in developing countries? Policy Research Department, World Bank, Washington, DC, USA. Policy Research Working Paper No. 1221.

Bloom, D.; Canning, D. 2000. The health and wealth of nations. Science, 287, 1207–1209.

Bosworth, B.; Collins, M. 1999. Capital flows to developing economies: implications for savings and investment. Brookings Papers on Economic Activity, 1 (spring), 143.

Boupha, B. 2000. The current status of health research capacity in Loa P.D.R. Paper presented at the WHO Meeting on Research Capacity Strengthening in Developing Countries, 26–28 Apr, Fondation Marcel Mérieux, Les Pensières, Annecy, France. World Health Organization, Geneva, Switzerland.

Bowles, S.; Gintis, H. 1996. Efficient redistribution: new rules for markets, states and communities. Politics and Society, 24(4), 307–342.

BRAC (Bangladesh Rural Advancement Committee). 2000. BRAC research 1999. BRAC, Dhaka, Bangladesh.

Braveman, P. 2000. Health inequalities and social inequalities in health [letter]. Bulletin of the World Health Organization, 78(2), 232–234.

Brown, K. 2000. A new breed of scientist–advocate emerges. Science, 287, 1192–1195.

Bruno, M.; Ravallion, M.; Squire, L. 1998. Equity and growth in developing countries: old and new perspectives on the policy issues. In Tanzi, V.; Chu, K., ed., Income distribution and high quality growth. Massachusetts Institute of Technology, Cambridge, MA, USA.

Buchanan, A. 1995. Privatization and just health care. Bioethics, 9, 220–239.

Burdach, E. 1998. Getting agencies to work together: the practice and theory of managerial craftsmanship. Brookings Institution Press, Washington, DC, USA.

Buse, K. 1999. Keeping a tight grip on the reins: donor control over aid coordination and management in Bangladesh. Health Policy and Planning, 14(3), 219–228.

Buse, K.; Walt, G. 2000a. Global public–private partnerships. Part 1: A new development in health? Bulletin of the World Health Organization, 78(4), 549–561.

———— 2000b. Global public–private partnerships. Part 2: What are the health issues for global governance? Bulletin of the World Health Organization, 78(5), 699–709.

Bush, K. 2000. Polio, war and peace. Bulletin of the World Health Organization, 78(3), 281–282.

Carr, D.; Gwatkin, D.; Fraqueiro, D.; Pande, R. 1999. A guide to country-level information about equity, poverty, and health available from multi-country research programs. World Bank, Washington, DC, USA.

Carrington, W.; Detragiache, E. 1999. How extensive is the brain drain? Finance and Development, 36(2), 46–49.

Castillo, G. 1993. Some thoughts on research capacity strengthening. ENHR Forum, 4(6), 2–3.

Castro-Leal, F.; Dayton, J.; Demery, L.; Mehra, K. 2000. Public spending on health care in Africa: do the poor benefit? Bulletin of the World Health Organization, 78(1), 66–74.

Cernea, M., ed. 1991. Putting people first: sociological variables in rural development. Oxford University Press, Oxford, UK.

Chalkley, K.; Shane, B. 1998. From research to action: how operations research is improving reproductive health services. Population Reference Bureau, United States Agency for International Development, Washington, DC, USA.

Chambers, R. 1983. Rural development: putting the last first. Longman, London, UK.

Chen, S.; Gaurav, D.; Ravallion, M. 1994. Is poverty increasing or decreasing in the developing world? Review of Income and Wealth, 40, 359–376.

Chongtrakul, P.; Okello, D. 2000. A manual for research priority setting using the ENHR strategy. Council on Health Research for Development, Geneva, Switzerland. Document No. 2000.3.

Choudhry, N.; Slaughter, P.; Sykora, K.; Naylor, C. 1997. Distributional dilemmas in health policy: large benefits for a few or smaller benefits for many? Journal of Health Services Research, 2(4), 212–216.

Choudhury, A.Y. 1999. Community participation in Essential National Health Research (ENHR) process: Bangladesh experience. Program for the Introduction and Adaptation of Contraceptive Technology, Bangladesh. Report for COHRED's Working Group on Community Participation.

CHRD (Commission on Health Research for Development). 1990. Health research: essential link to equity in development. Oxford University Press, New York, NY, USA.

CIHR (Canadian Institutes of Health Research). 2000. Where health research meets the future. CIHR, Ottawa, ON, Canada. Internet: http://www.cihr.org/

Clark, N. 1990. Development policy, technology assessment and the new technologies. Futures, 22(9), 913.

Coe, D.; Helpman, E.; Hoffmaister, A. 1997. North–South R&D spillovers (developing countries' benefits from industrial nations' research and development). Economic Journal, 107(440), 134–150.

Cohen, D. 1998. Managing knowledge in the new economy. The Conference Board, New York, NY, USA. Report 1222-98-CH.

COHRED (Council on Health Research for Development). 1993. Second International Conference on Health Research for Development, 8–9 March, Palais des Nations, Geneva, Switzerland. COHRED, Geneva, Switzerland.

——— 1994. Research capacity strengthening for Essential National Health Research (ENHR). COHRED, Geneva, Switzerland.
——— 1996. The next step: an interim assessment of ENHR and COHRED. COHRED, Geneva, Switzerland. Document No. 96.1.
——— 1997a. ENHR in Uganda: progress and challenges. COHRED, Geneva, Switzerland. Document No. 97.4.
——— 1997b. Essential National Health Research and priority setting: lessons learned. COHRED, Geneva, Switzerland. Document No. 97.3.
——— 1997c. Essential National Health Research in the Philippines: the first five years 1991-1996. COHRED, Geneva, Switzerland. Document No. 97.5.
——— 1998. Kampala workshop takes a critical look at district-level health research. COHRED Newsletter, 14, 5–9.
——— 1999. How to boost the impact of country mechanisms to support ENHR. A peek into the melting pot of country experiences. COHRED, Geneva, Switzerland. Document No. 99.1.
——— 2000a. Asian multi-country study on resource flows for health research and development. Report prepared by COHRED's Task Force on Resource Flows. COHRED, Geneva, Switzerland.
——— 2000b. Community participation in Essential National Health Research. Report of the Working Group on Community Participation, COHRED, Geneva, Switzerland. Document No. 2000.5.
——— 2000c. The ENHR handbook: a guide to Essential National Health Research. COHRED, Geneva, Switzerland. Document No. 2000.4.
——— 2000d. Equity issues back on the global agenda. COHRED Newsletter, 19, 2–3.
——— 2000e. Health research: powerful advocate for health and development based on equity. COHRED, Geneva, Switzerland. Document No. 2000.2.
——— 2000f. Working Group on Research to Action and Policy. COHRED, Geneva, Switzerland. Internet: http://www.cohred.ch
COHRED Newsletter. 1999. One decade of ENHR. COHRED Newsletter, 18, 9–12.
——— 2000. One decade of ENHR. COHRED Newsletter, 19, 10–14.
COHRED–WGPS (Council on Health Research for Development Working Group on Priority Setting). 2000. Priority setting for health research: lessons from developing countries. Health Policy and Planning, 15, 130–136.
Commission Secretariat. 1987. Independent International Commission on Health Research for Development (a planning meeting), 15–17 July, The Ecumenical Institute, Chateau de Bossey, Celigny, Switzerland. Harvard School of Public Health, Cambridge, MA, USA.
CONICYT (Comisión Nacional de Investigación Científica y Tecnológica–Chile). 1998. Annual report, 1998. CONICYT, Santiago, Chile.
Cornwall, A. 1996. Towards participatory practice: participatory rural appraisal (PRA) and the participatory process. *In* De Koning, K.;

Martin, M., ed., Participatory research in health: issues and experiences. Zed Press, London, UK.
Costello, A. 2000. A participatory approach to improve newborn care in Nepal. International Health Matters, 5, 10.

Das Gupta, M.; Aaby, P.; Pison, G.; Gareme, M., ed. 1997. Prospective community studies in developing countries. Clarendon Press, Oxford, UK.
Dasgupta, P.; David, P. 1994. Towards a new economics of science. Research Policy, 23, 487–521.
Davies, A.M.; Mansourian, B.P., ed. 1992. Research strategies for health: based on the Technical Discussions at the 43rd World Health Assembly on the Role of Health Research in the Strategy for Health for All by the Year 2000. Hogrefe and Huber Publishers, Lewiston, NY, USA.
De Koning, K.; Martin, M., ed. 1996. Participatory research in health: issues and experiences. Zed Press, London, UK.
Drucker, P. 1994. The age of social transformation. The Atlantic Monthly, Nov, pp. 53–80.

Estandarte, N.; Segovia, L.; Castillo, F.A. 2000. Sungki-sungking daan: lessons from NGO–Community Partnership for Women. Philippine Health Social Science Association, Manila, Philippines.
Evans, J. 1981. Measurement and management in medicine and health services: training needs and opportunities. The Rockefeller Foundation, New York, NY, USA.
Evans, T. 1989. The impact of permanent disability on rural households: river blindness in Guinea. IDS Bulletin, 20(2), 41–48.
Eyzaguirre, P. 1996. Agriculture and environmental research in small countries: innovative approaches to strategic planning. John Wiley and Sons, Chichester, UK.

Feachem, R. 2000. Poverty and inequity: a proper focus for the new century. Bulletin of the World Health Organization, 78(1), 1–2.
Fowler, A. 1997. Striking a balance: a guide to enhancing the effectiveness of non-governmental organizations in international development. Earthscan Publications Ltd, London, UK.
Francis, C.; Picou, D. 1999. Community participation in ENHR: Trinidad and Tobago. Report for COHRED's Working Group on Community Participation. Caribbean Health Research Council, Trinidad and Tobago.

Gadelha, C. 2000. Incorporating biotechnology research into health policy: the case of vaccine development and production in Brazil. Report prepared for COHRED's Working Group on Research to Policy; Oswaldo Cruz Foundation (Fiocruz), Brazil.
Gakidou, E.; Murray, C.; Frenk, J. 2000. Defining and measuring health inequality. Bulletin of the World Health Organization, 78(1), 42–54.

Garcia-Peñalosa, C. 1995. The paradox of education or the good side of inequality. Oxford Economic Papers, 47, 265–285.

Garrett, M.; Gransquist, C. 1998. Basic sciences and development: rethinking donor policy. Ashgate Publications, Brookfield, VT, USA.

GEOPS (Grupo de Estudios de Economía, Organización y Políticas Sociales). 1998. Priorities in collective health research in Latin America. GEOPS, Montevideo, Uruguay.

Gerhardus, A.; Kielman, K.; Sanou, A. 2000. The use of research for decision-making in the health sector. The case of "shared care" in Burkina Faso. Report prepared for COHRED's Working Group on Research to Policy, Department of Tropical Hygiene and Public Health, University of Heidelberg, Heidelberg, Germany; Nouna Centre for Health Research, Nouna, Burkina Faso.

GFHR (Global Forum for Health Research). 1999. The 10/90 report on health research 1999. GFHR, Geneva, Switzerland.

―――― 2000. The 10/90 report on health research 2000. GFHR, Geneva, Switzerland.

Gibbons, M.; Limoges, C.; Nowotny, H.; Schwartman, S.; Scott, P.; Trow, M. 1994. The new production of knowledge: the dynamics of science and research in contemporary societies. Sage Publications, London, UK.

Gibbs, W. 1995. Lost science in the Third World. Scientific American, 272(5), 92–99.

GON (Government of Norway). 1998. Institutional development in Norwegian bilateral assistance. Ministry of Foreign Affairs, Oslo, Norway. UD evaluation report 5.98.

Grabauskas, V. 2000. Health research profile: Lithuania (case study). Council on Health Research for Development, Geneva, Switzerland.

Guijt, I.; Shah, M.K., ed. 1998. The myth of community: gender issues in participatory development. Intermediate Technology Publications, London, UK.

Gwatkin, D. 2000. Health inequalities and the health of the poor: what do we know? What can we do? Bulletin of the World Health Organization, 78(1), 3–18.

Gwatkin, D.; Guillot, M. 2000. The burden of disease among the global poor: current situation, future trends, and implications for strategy. Global Forum for Health Research; Health, Nutrition and Population Department, World Bank, Washington, DC, USA.

Gwatkin, D.; Guillot, M.; Heuveline, P. 1999. The burden of disease among the global poor. The Lancet, 354, 586–589.

Haddad, S.; Fournier, P.; Machouf, N.; Yatara, F. 1998. What does quality mean to lay people? Community perceptions of PHC services in Guinea. Social Science and Medicine, 47, 381–394.

Halstead, S.; Tugwell, P.; Bennett, K. 1991. The International Clinical Epidemiology Network (INCLEN): a progress report. Journal of Clinical Epidemiology, 44, 579–589.

Hardon, A., ed. 1998. Beyond rhetoric: participatory research on reproductive health. Het Spinhuis, Amsterdam, Netherlands.
Harris, E. 1995. Working together: intersectoral action for health. Australian Government Publishing Service, Canberra, Australia.
Harrison, D. 1999. Social system intervention. In Perkins, E,; Simnett, I,; Wright, L., ed., Evidence based health promotion. John Wiley and Sons, New York, NY, USA. pp. 125–137.
——— 2000. Health research in Tanzania: how should the money be spent? Council on Health Research for Development, Geneva, Switzerland.
Harrison, D.; Neufeld, V. 2000. Capacity-building for health research in developing countries: no quick fix, but efforts could be boosted by greater efficiency. Council on Health Research for Development, Geneva, Switzerland. COHRED Working Paper.
Helpman, E. 1997. R&D and productivity: the international connection. National Bureau of Economic Research, Cambridge, MA, USA. NBER Working Paper 6101.4005897950.
Higginbotham, N. 1992. Developing partnerships for health and social science research: the International Clinical Epidemiology Network (INCLEN) Social Science Component. Social Science and Medicine, 35, 1325–1327.
Higginbotham, N.; Albrecht, G.; Connor, L. 2001. The new health social science: transdisciplinary perspective. Oxford University Press, Syndey, Australia.
Hilderbrand, M.; Grindle, M. 1994. Building sustainable capacity: challenges for the public sector. United Nations Development Programme, New York, NY, USA. Report on Project INT/92/676.
Horton, R. 2000. North and South: bridging the information gap. The Lancet, 355, 2231–2236.
HST (Health Systems Trust). 1999. South African health review 1999. HST, Durban, South Africa.
——— 2000. The equity gauge. HST, Durban, South Africa. Internet: http://www.hst.org.za/hlink/equity.htm

IDRC (International Development Research Centre). 1991. Final report: University Partnerships Project. IDRC, Ottawa, ON, Canada. Centre File 3-P-890-0184.
——— 1993. Future partnership for the acceleration of health development: report of a conference, 18–20 October 1993, Ottawa, Canada. IDRC, Ottawa, ON, Canada.
——— 1997. IDRC corporate program framework: to the year 2000. IDRC, Ottawa, ON, Canada, Mar.
IDRC; WHO (International Development Research Centre; World Health Organization). 1992. Managing health systems research. IDRC, Ottawa, ON, Canada; WHO, Geneva, Switzerland. Health Systems Research Training Series, Vol. 4.

ISDS (Initiative for Sub-District Support). 1998. The development of the district health system in South Africa: lessons learnt from the experience of ISDS. Health Systems Trust, Durban, South Africa. Technical Report 5. Internet: http://www.healthlink.org.za/hst/isds

Jareg, P.; Kaseje, D.C.O. 1998. Growth of civil society in developing countries: implications for health. The Lancet, 351, 819–822.
Jewkes, R.; Murcott, A. 1996. Meanings of community. Social Science and Medicine, 43(4), 555–563.
Johnson, B. 1994. The learning economy. Journal of Industry Studies, 1(2), 23–42.
Jones, C. 1995. R&D based models of economic growth. Journal of Political Economy, 103(4), 759–784.

Kawachi, I.; Kennedy, B. 1997. Socio-economic determinants of health: health and social cohesion: why care about income inequality? British Medical Journal, 314, 1037–1040.
Kawachi, I.; Kennedy, B.; Lochner, K.; Prothrow-Stith, D. 1997. Social capital, income inequality, and mortality. American Journal of Public Health, 87(9), 1491–1498.
Kennedy, B.; Kawachi, I.; Prothrow-Stith, D. 1996. Income distribution and mortality: cross-sectional ecological study of the Robin Hood Index in the United States. British Medical Journal, 312, 1004–1007.
Kholdy, S. 1995. Causality between foreign investment and spillover efficiency. Applied Economics, 27(8), 745–750.
Kickbush, I.; Quick, J. 1998. Partnerships for health in the 21st century. World Health Statistics Quarterly, 51, 68–74.
Kitua, A., ed. 1999. Tanzania Essential National Health Research Priority Setting Workshop. Arusha International Conference Center, Arusha, Tanzania, 15–21 Feb 1999. National Institute for Medical Research, Dar es Salaam, Tanzania.
Kuznets, S. 1955. Economic growth and income inequality. American Economic Review, 45, 1–28.

Lee, K. 1998. Shaping the future of global health cooperation: where can we go from here? The Lancet, 351, 899–902.
Lensink, R. 1996. Structural adjustment in sub-Saharan Africa. Longman, London, UK.
Loewenson, R. 1993. Structural adjustment and health policy in Africa. International Journal of Health Service, 23, 717–730.
Londoño, J.; Széleky, M. 1997. Persistent poverty and excess inequality: Latin America 1970–1995. Office of the Chief Economist, Inter-American Development Bank, New York, NY, USA. Working Paper Series 357.
Lucas, A. 1998. WHO at country level. The Lancet, 351, 743–47.

Lucas, A.; Mogedal, S.; Walt, G. 1997. Cooperation for health development: WHO's support to programmes at country level. London School of Hygiene and Tropical Medicine, London, UK.

Macfarlane, S.; Evans, T.; Muli-Musiime, F.; Prawl, O.; So, A. 2000. Global health research and INCLEN. The Lancet, 353, 503.

Mackenbach, J.; Kunst, A. 1997. Measuring the magnitude of socio-economic inequalities in health: an overview of available measures illustrated with two examples from Europe. Social Science and Medicine, 44(6), 757–771.

Makinen, M.; Waters, H.; Rauch M.; Almagambetova, N.; Bitran, R.; Gilson, L.; McIntyre, D.; Pannarunothai, S.; Prieto, A.; Ubilla, G.; Ram, S. 2000. Inequalities in health care use and expenditures: empirical data from eight developing countries and countries in transition. Bulletin of the World Health Organization, 78(1), 55–65.

Mansell, R; Wehn, U. 1998. Knowledge societies: information technology for sustainable development. Oxford University Press, New York, NY, USA.

Marmot, M.; Ryff, C.; Bumpass, L.; Shipley, M.; Marks, N. 1997. Social inequalities in health: next questions and converging evidence. Social Science and Medicine, 44(6), 901–910.

Marmot, M.G.; Shipley, M.J. 1996. Do socio-economic differences in mortality persist after retirement? 25 year follow-up of civil servants from the first Whitehall study. British Medical Journal, 313, 1177–1180.

McCoy, D. 1997. Health and health care in Mount Frere. Health Systems Trust, Durban, South Africa. Technical Report 2c. Internet: http://www.hst.org.za/isds

McDonald, S. 1998. Information for innovation: managing change from an information perspective. Oxford University Press, New York, NY, USA.

Mikkelsen, B. 1995. Methods for development work and research. Sage Publications India, New Delhi, India.

Miller, W.; Morris, L. 1999. 4th generation R&D: managing knowledge, technology and innovation. John Wiley and Sons, Inc., New York, NY, USA.

Misra, R. 1996. Using research findings: some Indian experiences. *In* Gwatkin, D.R., ed., How can research influence health policy? Reports from policymakers in three countries. International Health Policy Program, Washington, DC, USA. IHPP Occasional Paper, Feb.

Mooney, G. 1994. Key issues in health economics. Harvester Wheatsheaf, Hertfordshire, UK.

Morgan, L.M. 1993. Community participation in health: the politics of primary care in Costa Rica. Cambridge University Press, Cambridge, UK.

Murray, C.; Gakidou, E.; Frenk, J. 1999. Health inequalities and social group differences: what should we measure? Bulletin of the World Health Organization, 77(7), 537–543.

Nasseem, Z. 1992. African heritage and contemporary life: an experience of epistemological change. *In* McLean, G., ed., Cultural heritage and contemporary change. The Council for Research in Values and Philosophy, Washington, DC, USA. pp. 13–28. Series II: Africa. Vol. 2.

Navaretti, G.; Carraro, C. 1996. From learning to partnership: multinational R&D cooperation in developing countries. International Economics Department, World Bank, Washington, DC, USA. Policy Research Working Paper 1662.

Neema, S. 1999. Community participation in Essential National Health Research process: Uganda's experience. Report for COHRED's Working Group on Community Participation. Makerere Institute of Social Science, Makerere University, Uganda.

Nelson, R.; Winter, S. 1982. An evolutionary theory of economic change. Harvard University Press, Cambridge, MA, USA.

Neufeld, V.; Khanna, S.; Bramble, L.; Simpson, J. 1995. Leadership for change in the education of health professionals. Network Publications, Maastricht, Netherlands.

Ngwainmbi, G. 1999. Exporting communication technology to developing countries: socio-cultural, economic and educational factors. University Press of America, Inc., New York, NY, USA.

Nichter, M. 1984. Project community diagnosis: participatory research as a first step toward community involvement in primary health care. Social Science and Medicine, 19, 237–252.

NIMR (National Institute for Medical Research). 1999. Annual report. NIMR, Dar es Salaam, Tanzania.

Nooman, Z.M.; Mishriky, A.M. 1991. The Faculty of Medicine at Suez Canal University, Egypt. Teaching and Learning in Medicine, 3(4), 188–194.

Oakley, P. 1989. Community involvement in health development: an examination of the critical issues. World Health Organization, Geneva, Switzerland.

Ogunbode, O. 1991. Development of the Faculty of Health Sciences at the University of Ilorin, Nigeria. Teaching and Learning in Medicine, 3(4), 200–201.

Okello, D.; Emegu, P. 2000. Health research profile: Uganda. Council on Health Research for Development, Geneva, Switzerland.

Okurut, S. et al. 1996. Participatory research processes and empowerment: the PACODET community, Uganda. In de Koning, K.; Martin, M., ed., Participatory research in health: issues and experiences. Zed Press, London, UK.

Pang Soe, S.; Than Tuu, S. 2000. Research capacity strengthening for health development in Myanmar. Paper presented at the WHO Meeting on Research Capacity Strengthening in Developing Countries, 26–28 Apr, Fondation Marcel Mérieux, Les Pensières, Annecy, France. World Health Organization, Geneva, Switzerland.

Panisset, U. 1999. Latin American update. Presented at the Global Forum for Health Research. Forum 3, 8–10 Jun 1999. Global Forum for Health Research, Geneva, Switzerland. Doc 8.4.2.

Pavitt, K. 1991. What makes basic research economically useful? Research Policy, 20, 109–119.

Pegg, M. 1999. The art of mentoring. Management Books 2000 Ltd, Chalford, UK.

Pellegrini, A.; Amedia, N.; Trostle, J. 1998. Health research in Latin America and the Caribbean: tendencies and challenges. In Sanchez, D.; Bazzani, R.; Gomez, S., ed., Priorities in public health research in Latin America. Grupo de Estudios de Economía, Organización y Políticas Sociales, Montevideo, Uruguay.

Pereira, J. 1993. What does equity in health mean? Journal of Social Policy, 22(1), 19–48.

Persson, T.; Tabellini, G. 1994. Is inequality harmful for growth? American Economic Review, 84, 600–622.

Pfaff, W. 2000. The development numbers say economic globalism has failed. International Herald Tribune, 4 Jul.

Pfeffer, J.; Sutton, R. 2000. The knowing–doing gap: how smart companies turn knowledge into action. Harvard Business School Press, Boston, MA, USA.

Picou, D. 2000. Research and the health priority areas for the Caribbean. West Indies Medical Journal, 49(Suppl. 2), 1–2.

Pisano, G. 1991. The governance of innovation: vertical integration and collaborative arrangements in the biotechnology industry. Research Policy, 20, 237–249.

Porter, R. 1995. Knowledge utilization and the process of policy formulation: toward a framework for Africa. Support for Analysis and Research in Africa, Washington, DC, USA.

Pottier, J. 1997. Towards an ethnography of participatory appraisal and research. In Grillo, R.D.; Stirrat, R.L., ed., Discourses of development: anthropological perspectives. Berg, Oxford, UK.

Psacharopoulos, G. 1994. Returns to investment in education: a global update. World Development, 22(9), 1325–1343.

Putnam, R.; Leonardi, R.; Nanetti, R. 1993. Making democracy work. Civic traditions in modern Italy. Princeton University Press, Princeton, NJ, USA.

Ravallion, M. 1995. Growth and poverty: evidence from developing countries in the 1980s. Economic Letters, 48, 411–417.

———— 1997. Can high-inequality developing countries escape absolute poverty? Poverty and Human Resources Division, World Bank, Washington, DC, USA. Policy Research Working Paper 1775.

Ravallion, M.; Chen, S. 1997. What can new survey data tell us about recent changes in distribution and poverty? World Bank Economic Review, 11(2), 357–382.

Rebelo, S. 1998. The role of knowledge and capital in economic growth. World Institute for Development Economics Research, United Nations University, Helsinki, Finland. Working Paper No. 149.

Sachs, J. 1999. Helping the world's poorest. The Economist, 352(8132), 17.

―――― 2000. A new map of the world. The Economist (24 Jun), 81–83.

SARA (Support for Analysis and Research in Africa). 1997. Making a difference to policies and programs: a guide for researchers. SARA, Washington, DC, USA.

SAREC (Swedish Agency for Research Cooperation with Developing Countries). 1990. Karolinska Institute Nobel Conference – No 15. Health research for development. Stokholm, Sweden, 21–23 Feb 1990, SAREC, Stokholm, Sweden. SAREC Document. Conference Report 1990: 1

―――― 1995. Research for development: SAREC 20 years. SAREC, Stockholm, Sweden.

Schadler, S. 1996. How successful are IMF-supported adjustment programs? Finance and Development, 33 (Jun), 14–17.

Schultz, T. 1985. The economics of research and agricultural productivity. In Breth, S., ed., Five essays on science and farmers in the developing world. Winrock International Institute for Agricultural Development.

SCRPDC (Swiss Commission for Research Partnerships with Developing Countries). 1998. Guidelines for research in partnership with developing countries: 11 principles. SCRPDC, Bern, Switzerland.

Seeley, J.A.; Kengeya-Kayondo, J.F.; Mulder, D.W. 1992. Community-based HIV/AIDS research — whither community participation? Unsolved problems in a research programme in rural Uganda. Social Science and Medicine, 34(10), 1089–1095.

Segal, A. 1987. Learning by doing: science and technology in the developing world. Westview Press, Boulder, CO, USA.

Sen, A. 1992. Inequality reexamined. Russell Sage Foundation, New York, NY, USA.

―――― 1999a. Development as freedom. Alfred A. Knopf, New York, NY, USA.

―――― 1999b. Health and development. Bulletin of the World Health Organization, 77(8), 619–623.

Sen, B. 1999. Breaking the vicious circle of pverty using health. an analysis of possible routes. In Health in poverty reduction: collected papers. World Health Oganization, Geneva, Switzerland.

Shaw, R.; Elmendorf, A. 1994. Better health in Africa: experience and lessons learnt. World Bank, Washington, DC, USA.

SIDA–SAREC (Swedish International Development Agency–Swedish Agency for Research Cooperation with Developing Countries). 2000. Research co-operation. I: An outline of policy, programmes and practice. II: Trends in development. SIDA–SAREC, Stockholm, Sweden. Internet: http:/www.sida.se.

Silverstein, K. 1999. Millions for Viagra, pennies for diseases of the poor: research money goes to profitable lifestyle drugs. Nation, 269(3), 13.
Simon, J. 2000. Indicators for the measurement of research capacity strengthening investments. Paper presented at the WHO Meeting on Research Capacity Strengthening in Developing Countries, 26–28 Apr, Fondation Marcel Mérieux, Les Pensières, Annecy, France. World Health Organization, Geneva, Switzerland.
Sköld, M. 1999. Poverty and health: a global perspective. World Health Organization, Geneva, Switzerland.
Spiegel, P.; Salama, P. 2000. War and mortality in Kosovo, 1998–99: an epidemiological testimony. The Lancet, 355, 2204–2209.
Streeten, P. 1991. The impact of the changing world economy. *In* Singer, H.; Neelambar, H.; Rameshwar, T., ed., Joint ventures and collaborations. Indus Publishing Company, New Delhi, India.
Subbarao, K.; Bonnerjee, A.; Braithwaite, J.; Carvalho, S.; Ezemenari, K.; Graham, C.; Thompson, A. 1997. Safety net programs and poverty reduction: lessons from cross-country experience. World Bank, Washington, DC, USA.
Suwanwela, C. 1991. Strategy for change in an established medical school: a case study of the Faculty of Medicine at Chulalongkorn University, Thailand. Teaching and Learning in Medicine, 3(4), 210–214.
——— 2000. Health knowledge: the need for global cooperation. Paper presented at the Asia Forum for Health Research and Development, 17–19 Feb 2000, Manila, Philippines. Council on Health Research for Development, Manila, Philippines.
Sylla, N.D.; Diallo, A.A. 1999. Étude sur la participation communautaire dans la recherche essentielle en santé en République de Guinée [study of community participation in essential health research in Guinea]. Report for COHRED's Working Group on Community Participation. Ministry of Public Health, Guinea.

Tan, M.L.; Hardon, A. 1998. Particpatory research on reproductive health: introduction. *In* Hardon, A., ed., Beyond rhetoric: participatory research on reproductive health. Het Spinhuis, Amsterdam, Netherlands.
Tanzi, V.; Chu, K.; Gupta, S., ed. 1999. Economic policy and equity. International Monetary Fund, Washington, DC, USA.
Tarantola, D. 2000. Reducing HIV/AIDS risk, impact, and vulnerability. Bulletin of the World Health Organization, 78(2), 236–237.
TDR (Special Programme for Reseach and Training in Tropical Diseases). 1998. Final report: third external review. United Nations Develoment Programme; World Bank; World Health Organization; TDR, Geneva, Switzerland. TDR /JCB 921) 98.5.
Teece, D. 1987. Capturing value from technological innovation. In Guile, B.; Brooks, H., ed., Technology and global industry: companies and nations in the world economy. National Academy Press, Washington, DC, USA.

TEHIP News. 1999. Tanzania Health Intervention Project. TEHIP News, 1(1), 1–8.
Temple, J. 1999. The new growth evidence. Journal of Economic Literature, 37(1), 112–130.
TFHRD (Task Force on Health Research for Development). 1991. Essential National Health Research: a strategy for action in health and human development. TFHRD, Geneva, Switzerland.
Tobin, J. 1970. On limiting the domain of inequality. Journal of Law and Economics, 13(2), 263–277.
Tollman, S.M.; Zwi, A.B. 2000. Health system reform and the role of field sites based upon demographic and health surveillance. Bulletin of the World Health Organization, 78(1), 125–134.
Trostle, J.; Bronfman, M.; Langer, A. 1999. How do researchers influence decision-makers? Case studies of Mexican policies. Health Policy and Planning, 14(2), 103–114.

Ubel, P.; DeKay, M.; Baron, J.; Asch, D. 1996. Cost-effectiveness analysis in a setting of budget constraints. Is it equitable? New England Journal of Medicine, 334, 1174–1177.
UCD (Uganda Capacity Development ENHR Study Team). 1998. Capacity development for health research — a perspective from Uganda. COHRED Newsletter, 13, 1–4.
UNDP (United Nations Development Programme). 1996. UNDP's 1996 report on human development in Bangladesh: a pro-poor agenda. Orchid Printers, Dhaka, Bangladesh.
———— 1998. Capacity assessment and development: in a systems and strategic management context. Management Development and Governance Division, Bureau for Development Policy, UNDP, New York, NY, USA. Technical Advisory Paper No. 3.
———— 1999. Human development report 1999. Oxford University Press, New York, NY, USA.
———— 2000. Human development report 2000. Oxford University Press, New York, NY, USA
UNDP–TDR (United Nations Development Programme–World Bank–World Health Organization Special Programme for Research and Training in Tropical Diseases). 1999. WHO tropical disease research: progress 1997–98. Fourteenth programme report. World Health Organization, Geneva, Switzerland.
UNESCO (United Nations Educational, Scientific and Cultural Organization). 1999. Science and technology in Africa — a commitment to the 21st century. UNESCO, Paris, France. Internet: http://www/unesco.org/ope/scitech/facts.htm
Ustun, T. 2000. Mainstreaming mental health. Bulletin of the World Health Organization, 78(4), 412.

Wagstaff, A. 2000. Socioeconomic inequalities in child mortality: comparisons across nine developing countries. Bulletin of the World Health Organization, 78(1), 19–29.

Walrond, M. 1995. The Commonwealth Caribbean Medical Research Council, 1956–1995: a history. Commonwealth Caribbean Medical Research Council, Port of Spain, Trinidad.

Walt, G. 1994. Health policy. An introduction to process and power: people, governments and international agencies. Who drives policy and how it is made. Zed Books, London, UK.

Walt, G.; Pavignani, E.; Gilson, L.; Buse, K. 1999a. Health sector development: from aid coordination to resource management. Health Policy and Planning, 14(3), 207–218.

——— 1999b. Managing external resources in the health sector: are there lessons for SWAps? Health Policy and Planning, 14(3), 273–284.

Watkins, T. 1991. A technological communications costs model of R&D consortia as public policy. Research Policy, 20, 87–107.

Wayling, S. 1999. Assessment of TDR's research capability strengthening (RCS): 1990–1997. Paper presented to the Global Forum on Health Research, Jun 1999, Geneva, Switzerland.

Welch, F. 1999. In defense of inequality. American Economic Review Papers and Proceedings, 89, 226–242. Richard T. Ely Lecture.

White, K. 1991. Healing the schism: epidemiology, medicine, and the public's health. Springer-Verlag, New York, NY, USA.

Whitehead, M. 1992. The concepts and principles of equity and health. International Journal of Health Services, 22(3), 429–445.

WHO (World Health Organization). 1991. Strengthening research capabilities in the least developed countries. Report of a joint HRP, TDR, GPA consultation. WHO, Geneva, Switzerland. WHO/HRP/RIR/1991.

——— 1999. The world health report 1999: making a difference. WHO, Geneva, Switzerland.

——— 2000a. Health: a precious asset. WHO, Geneva, Switzerland. WHO/HSD/HID/00.1.

——— 2000b. WHO sets up high-level commission to study the links between health and economic growth. Bulletin of the World Health Organization, 78(2), 275.

——— 2000c. WHO Meeting on Research Capacity Strengthening (RCS) in Developing Countries. Report of the meeting held at Fondation Marcel Mérieux, Les Pensières, Annecy, France, 26–28 Apr, WHO, Geneva, Switzerland.

——— 2000d. The world health report 2000. Health systems: improving performance. World Health Organization, Geneva, Switzerland.

Wilkinson, R. 1992. Income distribution and life expectancy. British Medical Journal, 304, 165–168.

——— 1997. Commentary. Income inequality summarises the health burden of individual relative deprivation. British Medical Journal, 314, 1727–1728.

Willms, D.; Chingono, A.; Wellington, M.; Johnson, N. 1996. Designing an HIV/AIDS intervention for traditional healers in Zimbabwe. International Clinical Epidemiology Network, Philadelphia, PA, USA. Monograph No. 4. INCLEN Monograph Series on Critical International Health Issues.

Wolffers, I. 2000. Biomedical and development paradigms in AIDS prevention. Bulletin of the World Health Organization, 78(2), 267–273.

Wolffers, I.; Adjei, S.; van der Drift, R. 1998. Health research in the tropics. The Lancet, 351, 1652–1654.

Wolfson, M. 1994. When inequalities diverge. American Economic Review Papers and Proceedings, 84, 353–358.

World Bank. 1991. The African capacity building initiative: toward improved policy analysis and development management in sub-Saharan Africa. World Bank, Washington, DC, USA.

———— 1993. World development report 1993: investing in health. Oxford University Press, New York, NY, USA.

———— 1999. World development report 1998/99: knowledge for development. Oxford University Press, New York, NY, USA.

———— 2000. World development report 1999/2000: entering the 21st century. Oxford University Press, New York, NY, USA.

World Bank Group. 1997. Sector strategy: health, nutrition, and population. World Bank, Washington, DC, USA.

Yusuf, H.; Akhter, H.; Rahman, M.; Chowdhury, M.; Rochat, R. 2000. Injury-related deaths among women aged 10–50 years in Bangladesh, 1996–97. The Lancet, 355, 1220–1224.

Zakus, J.D.L.; Lysack, C.L. 1998. Revisiting community participation. Health Policy and Planning, 13(1), 1–12.

ABOUT THE INSTITUTION

The International Development Research Centre (IDRC) is committed to building a sustainable and equitable world. IDRC funds developing-world researchers, thus enabling the people of the South to find their own solutions to their own problems. IDRC also maintains information networks and forges linkages that allow Canadians and their developing-world partners to benefit equally from a global sharing of knowledge. Through its actions, IDRC is helping others to help themselves.

ABOUT THE PUBLISHER

IDRC Books publishes research results and scholarly studies on global and regional issues related to sustainable and equitable development. As a specialist in development literature, IDRC Books contributes to the body of knowledge on these issues to further the cause of global understanding and equity. IDRC publications are sold through its head office in Ottawa, Canada, as well as by IDRC's agents and distributors around the world. The full catalogue is available at http://www.idrc.ca/booktique.